GOUT DIET FOR DUMMIES

Most Effective Gout Diet Plan And Recipes To Lower Uric Acid Levels & Control Anti-Inflammatory Diseases

James C. Rutt

Table of content

INTRODUCTION

Gout is an arthritis that produces significant joint pain, edema, and inflammation. It is caused by high levels of uric acid in the blood. Uric acid is a waste product that is produced when the body breaks down purines. Purines are found in many foods, including organ meats, seafood, and beer.

A gout diet is one that contains less purines. This diet can help to reduce the amount of uric acid in the blood and help to prevent gout attacks. The diet should include plenty of low-purine foods, such as fruits, vegetables, whole grains, and low-fat dairy products.

If you suffer from gout, you may be all too familiar with the sudden, severe attacks of pain, swelling, redness and warmth in your joints. While there is no treatment for gout, dietary modifications might help prevent or alleviate its symptoms. A gout diet is typically low in purines, which are substances found in some foods and beverages that can contribute to gout.

Some foods that are high in purines include organ meats, such as liver and kidneys, as well as anchovies, herring, mackerel and other fatty fish. Other high-purine foods include dried beans and peas, beer and certain types of gravy.

While you don't need to eliminate these foods from your diet, you should limit your intake to avoid flare-ups. In addition, certain other foods and beverages can help prevent or relieve gout symptoms.

Cherries, for example, are often touted as a natural remedy for gout. Studies have shown that cherries, or cherry extract, can help to reduce the level of uric acid in the blood, which can help to prevent gout attacks.

Other foods that may be beneficial include complex carbohydrates, such as whole grains, and low-fat dairy products. These foods can help decrease uric acid levels in the blood by promoting its excretion.

Additionally, it is essential to maintain proper hydration by consuming a significant amount of water as well as other fluids. Drinking plenty of fluids helps to dilute the uric acid in the blood and helps to prevent its buildup.

While dietary changes can help prevent or relieve gout symptoms, it's important to talk to your doctor before making any drastic changes to your diet.

Millions of Americans suffer with gout and know how terrible it can be. But good news is, you can take care of your gout and get back to living a normal life. The most crucial step is to change your diet.

While there is no one-size-fits-all diet for gout, certain foods can help lower uric acid levels and reduce inflammation. This article will share the most effective gout diet plan and recipes to help you get started.

First, let's look at some gout-inducing foods. These include:

- Alcohol: Beer, wine, and liquor can all trigger gout flare-ups. Limit your alcohol consumption if you want to do so.

- Processed foods: Foods that are high in purines (a substance that breaks down into uric acid) can aggravate gout. Avoid processed meats, such as bacon, sausage, and lunch meats.

- Sugar-sweetened beverages: Soda, energy drinks, and fruit juices can all contribute to gout flare-ups. Drink just water or black tea and coffee without sugar.

- Refined carbs: White bread, pasta, and pastries can increase inflammation. Choose whole-grain options instead.

Now that you know which foods to avoid let's take a look at some of the best foods for gout. These include:

- Cherries: Cherries are rich in anthocyanins, which are compounds that reduce inflammation.

- Fatty fish: Fatty fish, such as salmon, mackerel, and tuna, are a good source of omega-3 fatty acids. These nutrients help to reduce inflammation.

- Broccoli: Broccoli is a nutrient-rich vegetable with antioxidants that help reduce inflammation.

-Green tea: Green tea is rich in polyphenols, compounds with anti-inflammatory properties.

- Apple cider vinegar: Apple cider vinegar helps to balance uric acid levels in the body.

Now that you know which foods to eat and avoid let's take a look at some gout-friendly recipes.

- Salmon and broccoli: This recipe is packed with anti-inflammatory nutrients. Simply bake or grill a piece of salmon, and serve it with steamed broccoli.

- Green tea and apple cider vinegar: This drink is a great way to start your day. Simply brew a cup of green tea and add a tbsp of apple cider vinegar.

-Tuna and brown rice: This recipe is an excellent source of omega-3 fatty acids. Cook brown rice according to package instructions. In a separate pan, cook tuna over medium heat. Once both components are cooked, combine them in a bowl.

-Cherry smoothie: This smoothie is a great way to get your daily dose of anthocyanins. Combine a cup of frozen cherries, a banana, and a cup of unsweetened almond milk in a blender and blend until smooth.

Following a gout diet can help to lower uric acid levels and reduce inflammation. There are many delicious recipes that you can enjoy while following this diet. By incorporating these foods into your diet, you can help to manage your gout and get your life back.

1. PUMPKIN BAKED OATMEAL

Prep Time: 15 Mins

Cook Time: 30 Mins

Total Time: 45 Mins

Servings: 6

Ingredients

- 2 cups of old-fashioned rolled oats
- 1 tsp baking powder
- 1 ½ tsp pumpkin pie spice
- ½ tsp cinnamon
- ½ tsp sea salt
- 1 ½ cups of unsweetened almond milk
- 1 cup of canned pumpkin
- ¼ cup of pure maple syrup + more for serving
- 1 tbsp ground flaxseed
- 1 tbsp coconut oil melted
- 1 tsp vanilla extract
- ½ cup of pecans or walnuts chopped and divided
- Cooking spray

Instructions

1. Heat the oven to 375°F.
2. Cooking spray an 8-inch square baking pan.
3. Combine the oats, baking powder, pumpkin pie spice, cinnamon, and salt in a large mixing bowl. To combine, stir everything together.
4. Combine the milk, pumpkin, maple syrup, flaxseed, coconut oil, and vanilla in a bowl. Stir well to incorporate, then add ¼ cup of pecans or walnuts gradually.
5. Carefully pour the oatmeal mixture into the pan.
6. Spread the remaining pecans or walnuts on top.

7. 30–35 minutes, until golden and set. Take it from the oven and set it aside for a few minutes to cool. Serve in portions. Drizzle maple syrup over each serving if you want it sweeter.
8. Refrigerate it in an airtight jar for up to 4 days.
9. To reheat the entire baked oatmeal, cover with foil and bake at 350°F for about 20 minutes. Set the oven (or toaster oven) to 350°F and bake for 5-10 minutes for individual servings, or reheat in microwave for 1 minute.

2. MINI FRUIT TARTS WITH VANILLA PASTRY CREAM

Prep Time: 45 Mins

Cook Time: 45 Mins

Chill Time: 3 Hrs

Total Time: 4 Hrs 30 Mins

Servings: 13 -14

Ingredients

Mini-Tart Crust

- 1½ cups of unbleached flour
- ⅓ cup of powdered sugar
- ¼ tsp salt
- ½ cup of chilled butter
- 1 egg yolk
- 1 tbsp heavy cream

Cream Filling:

- 2¾ cups of milk
- ⅔ cup of sugar
- ¼ cup of cornstarch
- ⅛ tsp salt
- 4 egg yolks
- 2 tbsp of butter
- 1 tsp vanilla extract

Glaze

- ¼ cup of currant jelly

Instructions

Crust

1. In a food processor, combine 1 ½ cups of flour, ⅓ cup of sugar, and ¼ tsp of salt.
2. ½ cup of butter, cut into 8 pieces, add to flour mixture, pulsing several times until mixture resembles oatmeal 1 egg yolk and 1 tbsp of cream.
3. Mix until all the ingredients are moistened. Let the machine run for just a few seconds or until the dough begins to stick together. (You may add a few more drops of milk or cream if the dough seems dry.)
4. Roll the dough out like chilled cookie dough. Warp with plastic wrap and put in the refrigerator for 30 minutes.
5. Spray the molds liberally with Baker's Secret or something like. (Baker's Secret is a flour-and-oil aerosol spray.) Greasing is not required when using silicone molds.
6. Cut the dough roll into 12 pieces. Roll the dough between two pieces of plastic wrap into a circle slightly bigger than the tart shapes. With your fingers, press into a mold, being careful to keep the thickness consistent. Trim any excess at the top using a knife. Refrigerate for 30 minutes minimum and up to one month. Line a cookie sheet with frozen tart shells. Insert a tiny square of foil into each crust and shape it to fit the form of the crust.
7. Bake for 10 minutes at 400°F. Remove foil and bake 3-4 minutes, or until the food is golden brown.

Cream Filling

8. Add 2 ¾ c milk, ⅔ c sugar, ¼ c cornstarch, ⅛ t salt, and 4 egg yolks, to a mixer or food processor bowl. (You can use a bowl and a mixing bowl if that is all you have.)
9. After 5 seconds, put into a 2-quart glass microwave-safe mixing bowl.
10. Microwave on high for 6-7 minutes, mixing every 3 minutes until smooth. (If the mixture is still thick after 7 minutes, continue to microwave.)
11. Whisk in 2 tbsp butter and 1 tsp vanilla extract until smooth.
12. Cover the top of the heated custard with plastic wrap and smooth it to touch the surface if not ready to assemble. This keeps the cream from getting a skin on top.

Assembly

13. Fill each cooked tart shell with cream filling. Top with your favorite fruit.

Glaze

14. Melt ¼ cup of currant jelly in the microwave or on the stove and dab some shine on every piece of fruit using a brush. It is OK if some spills onto the cream.

Notes

1. If it appears too dry to form into a ball, add a tsp or two of milk or cream to the dough in the food processor.
2. Tarts are best consumed on the day they are made.
3. These are even better with a dollop of whip cream.

3. PARMALET (CRISP PARMESAN OMELET)

Prep Time: 10 Mins

Cook Time: 5 Mins

Total Time: 15 Mins

Servings: 1

Ingredients

- 2 eggs
- ¼ tsp water
- 1 tsp olive oil
- Toss with freshly ground black pepper and kosher salt to taste
- 1 ounce of freshly grated Parmigiano-Reggiano cheese, or a little less
- 1 pinch of cayenne pepper

Instructions

1. In a mixing bowl, crack the eggs. ¼ tsp of water and stir until just combined (do not overmix).
2. In an 8-inch nonstick pan, sprinkle olive oil. Brush the bottom of the pan equally. Grate the cheese into the pan equally, about ½-inch deep (or just shy of 1 ounce).
3. Heat the pan on medium-high. The cheese will begin to melt gradually. Pour eggs evenly over cheese as it begins to bubble and turn golden brown, around 4 minutes. Turn the heat down low. Sprinkle with salt, pepper, and cayenne pepper. Cook the eggs on low heat until they are set, checking every 30 seconds. This should take around 1 minute of total cooking time for 2 eggs.

4. Remove the pan from the heat. Fold the parmalat in half carefully using a spatula. Place it on a serving plate.

4. BANANA PANCAKES

Total Time: 20 Mins

Servings: 4

Ingredients

For pancakes

- 1½ cups of all-purpose flour spooned into measuring cup and leveled off
- 2 tbsp of sugar
- 2½ tsp of baking powder
- ½ tsp salt
- 1 small, over-ripe banana, peeled (the browner, the better)
- 2 large eggs
- 2 tbsp plus 1 cup of low-fat milk
- ½ tsp vanilla extract
- 3 tbsp of melted unsalted butter

For cooking

- 1-2 tbsp of vegetable oil
- 1 tbsp unsalted butter
- **For serving**
- Maple syrup
- Sliced bananas
- Confectioners' sugar (optional)

Instructions

1. First, blend flour, sugar, baking powder, and salt in a medium bowl.
2. Smash the banana with a fork in a small bowl until nearly smooth. Mix in the eggs, then the milk and vanilla extract until completely combined. Combine the banana mixture with the melted butter in a mixing bowl. Fold the batter carefully with a

rubber spatula until just incorporated; do not over-mix. The batter will be lumpy and thick.

3. Heat a griddle pan over medium heat. Stir a pad of butter and one tbsp of vegetable oil on the griddle. Drop the batter onto the griddle by 14 cup of fuls, spacing the pancakes approximately 2 inches apart. Cook for 2 minutes until a few holes appear on top of each pancake and the bottom is golden brown. Cook the pancakes for another 1 to 2 minutes, until the bottom, is golden brown and the top is puffed. Transfer the pancakes to a serving platter using a spatula.

4. Wipe off the griddle with paper towels, then add additional butter and oil and repeat with the leftover batter. If preferred, serve the pancakes hot with maple syrup, chopped bananas, and confectioners' sugar.

5. ARANCINI

Prep Time: 1 Hr 50 Mins

Cook Time: 40 Mins

Total Time: 2 Hr 30 Mins

Servings: 4

Ingredients

- 3 cups of low-sodium chicken broth
- Kosher salt
- 1 cup of arborio rice
- 2 tbsp toasted pine nuts
- ½ cup of shredded mozzarella cheese
- ½ cup of shredded fontina cheese
- 2 tbsp chopped fresh parsley
- 2 large eggs
- ½ cup of grated parmesan cheese
- 1 ½ cups of breadcrumbs
- Vegetable oil for frying

Instructions

1. Bring the broth and ¼ tsp of salt to a boil in a medium saucepan over medium-high heat. Mix in the rice, lower to a low heat, and cook until soft, about 20 minutes. Allow to cool fully on a baking sheet lined with parchment paper.
2. Set aside the pine nuts, mozzarella, fontina, and parsley in a bowl.
3. In a large bowl, mix the eggs, cooled rice, parmesan, and ⅔ cup of breadcrumbs. Form the mixture into sixteen 1 ½ -inch balls.
4. In a shallow bowl, combine the remaining breadcrumbs. Insert 2 tbsp of the mozzarella mixture into the middle of each rice ball, then crimp the rice around the filling to enclose. Roll the balls in the breadcrumbs and arrange them on a baking sheet lined with parchment paper. Lid loosely and refrigerate for a minimum of 1 hour or overnight. (If chilling overnight, roll in more breadcrumbs before frying.)
5. In a large saucepan, heat ½ inch vegetable oil over medium heat until a deep-fry thermometer reads 350 °F. Fry the rice balls in batches, rotating once, until golden brown on all sides, about 4 minutes. Drain on paper towels after taking with a slotted spoon.

6. EASY OVERNIGHT OATS

Total Time: 5 Mins

Servings: 1

Ingredients

Base

- ½ cup of old-fashioned rolled oats
- ½ cup of milk of choice
- ¼ cup of non-fat Greek yogurt
- 1 tbsp chia seeds
- 1 tbsp sweetener, honey or maple syrup
- ¼ tsp vanilla extract

Peanut Butter & Jelly

- 1 tbsp strawberry jam
- 1 tbsp creamy peanut butter
- ¼ cup of diced strawberries
- 2 tbsp crushed peanuts

Apple Pie

- ¼ cup of diced apples
- 1 tbsp of chopped pecans
- 2 tsp maple syrup
- ¼ tsp cinnamon

Banana Nutella

- ½ banana sliced
- 1 tbsp Nutella
- 1 tbsp crushed hazelnuts
- 1 tbsp chips chocolate

Almond Joy

- ¼ cup of shredded coconut
- 1 tbsp chopped almonds
- 1 tbsp chips chocolate
- 2 tsp maple syrup

Instructions

1. In a large glass jar, mix all of the ingredients until thoroughly incorporated.
2. Use a cover or plastic wrap to protect the glass container. Refrigerate for 2 hours or overnight. Toppings can be added the day before or right before serving.
3. The next day, remove the lid and serve from the glass container. If necessary, thin with a bit more milk or water.

Notes

1. Overnight oats can be kept in the fridge for up to 5 days. This makes it a great Sunday night breakfast meal preparation for the week.
2. **Make it vegan:** Sweeten with plant-based milk, plant-based yogurt, and maple syrup.
3. **Make it gluten-free:** Make use of gluten-free oats.
4. To make it sugar-free, leave out the sweetener entirely or replace it with mashed or pureed fruit in the base recipe.

7. ZUCCHINI FRITTATA

Prep Time: 10 Mins

Bake Time: 20 To 25 Mins

Total Time: 1 Hr 50 Mins

Servings: one 9" or 10" round frittata

Ingredients

- 6 cups of grated zucchini, or summer squash
- ½ tsp salt
- 1 large peeled and diced sweet onion
- 1 ½ cups of Parmesan cheese
- 8 large eggs
- 2 tbsp of All-Purpose Flour or 2 tbsp of Gluten-Free All-Purpose Flour

Instructions

1. Mix the salt into the shredded squash. Put the squash in a colander, weigh it down, and drain for about an hour.
2. Combine the drained squash and onion in a bowl. Fry the veggies in 2 tbsp of olive oil in a large pan until tender, around 20 minutes; the volume will be greatly reduced. Add more salt and pepper to taste.
3. Preheat the oven to 400 degrees Fahrenheit.
4. In a big bowl, mix the cheese, eggs, and flour.
5. Drain any excess liquid from the cooked squash. To combine, stir everything together.
6. 1 tbsp olive oil in a 9" or 10" cast iron skillet, heat until the oil is extremely hot.
7. In the pan, evenly distribute the vegetable mixture. Bake, the frittata for 20 to 25 minutes, or until the top is light golden brown.

8. Take them from the oven and serve immediately in wedges.

8. GRILLED POTATOES WITH BACON-RANCH SAUCE

Total Time: 30 Mins

Servings: 5

Ingredients

- 2 tbsp olive oil
- 1 tbsp barbecue seasoning
- 2 garlic cloves, minced
- 2 tsp lemon juice
- 1- ½ pounds small potatoes, quartered

Sauce

- ⅔ cup of ranch salad dressing
- 4 tsp bacon bits
- 2 tsp minced chives
- Dash hot pepper sauce

Instructions

1. Mix the oil, barbecue spice, garlic, and lemon juice in a large bowl. Toss in the potatoes to coat. Place a second layer of heavy-duty foil on top (about 28 in. square). Fold the foil around the potato mixture and seal tightly.
2. Cook, covered, over medium heat for 20-25 minutes, or until potatoes are soft.
3. Combine the sauce ingredients in a small bowl. Serve with mashed potatoes.

9. HONEY SOY CHICKEN STIR FRY

Prep Time: 10 Mins

Cook Time: 20 Mins

Total Time: 30 Mins

Servings: 4

Ingredients

- 1 tbsp vegetable oil
- 1 pound of skinless, boneless chicken breasts, sliced into 1" pieces
- 2 tsp minced ginger
- 2 zucchini, quartered and sliced
- 1 red bell pepper, peeled and seeded, cut into 1-inch pieces
- ¼ cup of low-sodium chicken broth
- ¼ cup of low sodium soy sauce
- 3 tbsp of honey
- salt and pepper to taste
- 2 tbsp sliced green onions
- 2 tsp cornstarch

Instructions

1. Heat the oil in a big pan over medium-high heat. Sprinkle the chicken to taste with salt and pepper.
2. Cook the chicken in a single layer in the pan until brown. You might have to work in bunches.
3. After add the ginger to the chicken, cook for 30 seconds additional.
4. To keep the chicken mixture warm, place it on a platter and cover it with foil.
5. Cook until the zucchini and red bell pepper are tender, about 3 to 4 minutes. Return the chicken to the pan with the veggies.
6. In a bowl, combine the chicken broth, honey, and soy sauce.
7. Combine the cornstarch and a tbsp of cold water in a small bowl.
8. Cook for 30 seconds after pouring the chicken broth mixture over the chicken and veggies.
9. Add the cornstarch and cook for one minute or until the sauce thicken.
10. Serve garnished with green onions.

10. LEMON & HERB MUSHROOM BRUSCHETTA

Prep Time: 10 Mins

Cook Time: 15 Mins

Total Time: 25 Mins

Servings: 4

Ingredients

- 1 tbsp olive oil
- 2 tbsp of unsalted butter
- 200g sliced brown mushrooms
- 1 crushed garlic clove
- 1 tsp lemon zest
- 1 tbsp lemon juice
- 1 tsp of fresh thyme leaves
- 1 tbsp parsley leaves
- Salt and pepper to season

To serve

- Shaved parmesan cheese
- Rocket leaves
- A crusty loaf of sliced bread

Instructions

1. For a minute, heat the olive oil, butter, and garlic in a skillet over medium heat. Add the mushrooms and cook for approximately five minutes.
2. Cook for another five minutes, or until the liquid begins to evaporate, with the lemon juice, lemon zest, and thyme leaves.
3. Take it from the heat and season with salt and pepper to taste. Incorporate chopped parsley.
4. Toast one piece of bread. Add a handful of rocket leaves, sautéed mushrooms, and shaved parmesan cheese on top.

11. AVOCADO TOAST

Prep Time: 3 Mins

Cook Time: 2 Mins

Total Time: 5 Mins

Servings: 1

Ingredients

- 1 slice of bread
- ½ ripe avocado
- Pinch of salt
- Any of the extra toppings are optional

Instructions

1. Bake your bread until it is brown and firm.
2. Take off the pit of your avocado. Scoop the flesh out using a large spoon. Mash it with a fork in a bowl until it's as smooth as you want it. Mix with a pinch of salt (approximately ⅛ tsp) and adjust to taste.
3. On top of your bread, spread avocado.

12. PEANUT BUTTER ACAI BOWL

Prep Time: 5 Mins

Total Time: 5 Mins

Servings: 1

Ingredients

- 1½ peeled and frozen bananas
- ½ cup of frozen strawberries
- ½ cup of frozen blueberries
- 100g frozen unsweetened acai blend
- 2 heaping tbsp of creamy peanut butter
- ¼ cup of milk of choice
- Toppings (such as granola, berries, and peanut butter)

Instructions

1. Mix the bananas, berries, acai berry package, peanut butter, and milk of choice in a high-powered blender. Blend on high until totally smooth.
2. Garnish with granola, berries, and a drizzle of peanut butter in a bowl. Enjoy right now.

13. GUACAMOLE SANDWICH RECIPE

Prep Time: 10 Mins

Cook Time: 10 Mins

Total Time: 20 Mins

Servings: 4

Ingredients

- Measuring cup used 1 cup

For Guacamole

- 3 medium avocados ripened
- ½ cup of finely chopped red onions
- ½ large chopped roma tomato seeds and pulp removed, (optional)
- ½ large jalapeno finely chopped or serrano peppers
- 2 tbsp of cilantro (coriander leaves)
- 2 tbsp of fresh lime juice
- salt and black pepper to taste

For Sandwich

- 8 bread slices
- Cheese optional
- 2-3 tbsp of butter or oil to toast

Instructions

Making the guacamole:

1. Mash the avocados with a fork or a potato masher in a mixing bowl to the desired consistency.

2. Mix in the onions, jalapeo, cilantro, lime juice, salt, and black pepper until thoroughly combined. (If using tomatoes, add them at the end since they release moisture.)

For the Sandwich:

3. Heat a tawa over medium heat. Toast the bread on both edges with butter or oil until golden brown and crunchy.
4. Arrange the toasted bread on a plate to serve.
5. Spread 2 to 3 tbsp of guacamole on the bread piece, then top with another bread slice.
6. Cut it in half and immediately serve with a cup of tea or coffee.

14. HUEVOS RANCHEROS BREAKFAST SANDWICH

Prep Time: 5 Mins

Cook Time: 5 Mins

Total Time: 10 Mins

Servings: 2

Ingredients

- 2 english muffins, halved and toasted
- ⅓ cup of refried beans
- 2 eggs
- 1 Avocado
- Salsa
- Salt and Pepper

Instructions

1. While the english muffins toast, peel and pit the California Avocado and mash it with a fork. Season with salt to taste. Microwave refried beans until warm and spreadable. Distribute half of the bean mixture on each English muffin's bottom, then spread half of the avocado on each top.
2. Melt butter in a mini nonstick pan over medium-high heat. Apply olive oil to the pan. Crack eggs and place them, one by one, in the pan, ensuring sure the egg whites do not touch. Season with salt and pepper to taste. Allow 1-2 minutes, or longer if

preferred, before carefully flipping the eggs over with a spatula. Sprinkle with salt once more. Cook for about 1-2 minutes, or until done. Put the cooked egg on top of the beans on the English muffin. Repeat with the other egg.

3. Place the egg on top of the salsa, then top with the avocado-smeared side of the english muffin. Enjoy!

15. EGG SANDWICHES WITH ROSEMARY, TOMATO & FETA

Prep Time: 5 Mins

Cook Time: 15 Mins

Total Time: 20 Mins

Servings: 4

Ingredients

- 4 multigrain sandwich thins
- 4 tsp olive oil
- 1 tbsp snipped fresh rosemary or ½ tsp dried rosemary, crushed
- 4 eggs
- 2 cups of fresh baby spinach leaves
- 1 medium tomato, peeled and cut into 8 thin slices
- 4 tbsp of reduced-fat feta cheese
- ⅛ tsp kosher salt
- freshly ground black pepper

Instructions

1. Preheat the oven to 375 °F. Brush the cut sides of the sandwich thins with 2 tbsp of olive oil. Place on a baking pan and toast for 5 minutes, or until the edges are light golden and crunchy.
2. Meanwhile, in a big skillet over medium-high heat, sauté the remaining 2 tbsp of olive oil and rosemary. One at a time, crack the eggs into the pan. Cook for 1 minute, or until the whites are firm but the yolks are still runny. Using a spatula, break the yolks. Cook until the eggs are done on the other side. Turn off the heat.
3. Place the toasted sandwich thin bottom halves on four serving plates. Place spinach between the sandwich thins on the plates. Top each with two tomato slices, an egg, and one tbsp of feta cheese. Season with salt and pepper to taste. Place the remaining sandwich thin halves on top.

16. ZUCCHINI BANANA MUFFINS

Prep Time: 20 Mins

Cook Time: 20 Mins

Total Time: 40 Mins

Servings: 14

Ingredients

- 2 cups of all-purpose flour
- 1 tsp baking powder
- 1 tsp baking soda
- ½ tsp salt
- ½ tsp ground cinnamon
- ⅓ cup of canola, or vegetable oil
- ¾ cup of packed light brown sugar
- 1 ½ cups of pureed ripe banana
- 2 tsp of vanilla extract
- 2 large eggs, room temperature
- 1 cup of grated zucchini
- Banana chips, optional

Instructions

1. Preheat oven to 425°F. Coat or line 14 muffin cups with cooking spray; put aside.
2. Combine the flour, baking powder, baking soda, salt, and powdered cinnamon in a large mixing basin. To combine, mix everything together. Make a well in the middle and set it aside.
3. Mix together the oil, sugar, banana, and vanilla in a separate bowl or large liquid measuring cup until thoroughly combined. Stir in the eggs to mix. Incorporate the zucchini.
4. Fill the middle of the dry ingredients with the mixture. Fold the batter with a silicone spatula until the dry ingredients are moistened.
5. Add about two-thirds of the batter to each muffin cup that has been prepped. If desired, top each with a banana chip.
6. 5 minutes in the oven. When a wooden pick put into the centre comes out clean, lower the oven temperature to 350 degrees Fahrenheit and simmer for another 10

to 15 minutes. Take care not to overbake the muffins, as this may cause them to dry out.

7. Take the muffins from the pan and set them aside for 10 minutes before serving.

17. GLUTEN-FREE PANCAKES

Prep Time: 5 Mins

Cook Time: 25 Mins

Total Time: 30 Mins

Servings: 6 small pancakes

Ingredients

- 125g gluten-free plain flour
- 1 egg
- 250ml milk
- butter, for frying

Instructions

1. To begin, place the flour in a bowl and make a well in the middle. Crack the egg in the center and add a quarter of the milk. Utilize an electric or balloon whisk to blend the ingredients well. Once you have a paste, add another quarter and, once lump-free, the remaining milk. Allow for a 20-minute rest. Stir once more before using.
2. In a small nonstick frying pan, melt a knob of butter. When the butter begins to froth, pour a tiny bit of the mixture into the pan and swirl around to coat the bottom-a thin coating is fine. Cook for a few minutes until the bottom is golden brown, then flip and cook until the other side is golden. Repeat until all batter is consumed, stirring it between pancakes and adding more butter to the pan as required.
3. Garnish with agave syrup and an orange juice squeeze, or with your favorite pancake filling.

18. CINNAMON WAFFLES - EASY AND DELICIOUS!

Prep Time: 10 Mins

Cook Time: 4 Mins

Total Time: 14 Mins

Servings: 4

Ingredients

- 1 ¾ cups of milk
- ½ cup of oil
- 1 tsp vanilla
- 2 eggs
- 2 cups of flour
- 4 tsp baking powder
- ½ tsp salt
- 2 tbsp of sugar
- 2 tsp of cinnamon

Instructions

1. In a small bowl, add the flour, baking powder, sugar, salt, and cinnamon. In a medium bowl, mix the milk, oil, vanilla, and eggs using a mixer.
2. Mix the wet and dry ingredients together until just mixed (a few small lumps are okay). Allow for a five-minute rest.
3. Preheat your waffle iron while the batter rests. Cook according to the waffle maker's directions. (One cup of dough cooked for four minutes in my Belgian waffle maker was great.)
4. If preferred, serve it warm with syrup, whipped cream, and cinnamon on top.

19. CHEESE GRIT-AND-CHIVE MUFFINS

Prep Time: 15 Mins

Cook Time: 30 Mins

Total Time: 45 Mins

Servings: 2

Ingredients

- Butter
- 1 ½ cups of all-purpose flour
- 1 tsp baking powder
- ½ tsp baking soda
- ½ tsp kosher salt
- 2 large eggs
- ¾ cup of buttermilk
- ½ cup of melted butter
- 1 cup of cooked grits
- 1 cup of grated sharp Cheddar cheese
- 1 tbsp chopped fresh chives
- Ground red pepper

Instructions

1. Preheat the oven to 350 degrees. Grease 24 small muffin cups lightly with butter.
2. Combine flour and the next 3 ingredients in a large bowl. Mix the eggs, buttermilk, and melted butter in a separate bowl. Add grits to the egg mixture and stir. Stir the grit mixture into the flour mixture. Mix the cheese, chives, and ground red pepper to taste.
3. Pour roughly three-fourths of the batter into each muffin cup. Bake for 30–35 minutes, or until the muffins are golden brown and separate from the pan's sides.

20. CHAI SPICED BREAKFAST QUINOA

Prep Time: 5 Mins

Cook Time: 25 Mins

Total Time: 25 Mins

Servings: 2

Ingredients

- 2 cups of almond milk, plus more for serving
- 1 cup of dry quinoa
- ½ tsp ground cinnamon
- ¼ tsp ground ginger
- 1 pinch cloves
- 1 pinch cardamom
- 1 pinch salt
- 2 tbsp of honey, or to taste
- ¼ tsp vanilla extract, optional

Instructions

1. Bring almond milk, cinnamon, ginger, cloves, cardamom, and salt to a boil in a medium saucepan. Lower the heat and stir in the quinoa.
2. Cover and simmer for 15 to 20 minutes until the almond milk has been absorbed, and the quinoa is cooked.
3. Mix in the honey and vanilla extract. Serve warm, topped with more almond milk.

21. BREAKFAST PARFAIT WITH GREEK YOGURT, FRESH BERRIES, AND GRANOLA

Total Time: 7 Mins

Servings: 2

Ingredients

- 5.3-ounce plain Greek yogurt
- ½ small sliced banana
- 4 to 5 fresh sliced strawberries
- 15 fresh blueberries
- 6 raspberries
- 1 to 2 tbsp classic granola

Instructions

1. Spread yogurt on the bottom of a large soup or pasta bowl.
2. Layer each fruit in a row, beginning with strawberries, then blueberries, banana slices, then raspberries.
3. Sprinkle granola around the bowl with a spoonful.
4. Serve right away.

22. BLACK BEAN SCRAMBLE

Prep Time: 6 Mins

Cook Time: 7 Mins

Total Time: 13 Mins

Servings: 1

Ingredients

- 2 eggs
- ¼ tsp ground cumin
- Dash of garlic salt
- Dash of freshly ground black pepper
- ¼ cup of drained and rinsed black beans
- 1 tbsp purchased chunky salsa
- ¼ cup of shredded Mexican cheese

Instructions

1. Set aside the eggs, cumin, garlic salt, and pepper to mix together.
2. Cook, often turning, for around 30 seconds, until the salsa liquid has evaporated in a small nonstick pan over medium-high heat.
3. Mix the egg mixture into the skillet until the eggs are nearly done.
4. Continue to cook, stirring, until the eggs achieve the desired consistency.
5. Place to a platter and top with the remaining cheese before serving.

23. BREAKFAST EGG MUFFINS WITH PEPPER AND GREEN ONION

Prep Time: 15 Mins

Cook Time: 20 Mins

Total Time: 35 Mins

Servings: 6

Ingredients

- 6 eggs
- ¼ cup of grated cheddar cheese
- ½ diced red pepper
- 1 green onion
- ¼ tsp olive oil

Instructions

1. Turn the oven on to 375°F.
2. In a nonstick skillet, heat the oil. Add the pepper, green onion, and sauté for 2 to 3 minutes, or until just starting to soften.
3. Using a little oil and some kitchen paper, grease the cups a nonstick, 6 muffin pan.
4. In a small bowl, crack one of the eggs and mix it to mix.
5. Pour into the muffin tin and continue with the remaining eggs to fill each of the 6 muffin cups.
6. Add salt and pepper to taste.
7. Then, evenly distribute the cooked veggies among the muffin cups.
8. Incorporate the cheese into each muffin cup after evenly distributing it.
9. 20 minutes of baking or until the tops are firm.

24. ALMOND OAT PANCAKES

Prep Time: 10 Mins

Cook Time: 5 Mins

Total Time: 15 Mins

Servings: 10

Ingredients

- 1 cup of almond flour
- 1 cup of oat flour
- ½ tsp baking soda
- ½ tsp baking powder
- ½ tsp salt
- ½ tsp cinnamon
- 2 tbsp of maple syrup
- 2 eggs
- 2 tbsp melted butter
- 1 cup of milk

Instructions

1. In a bowl, mix almond flour, oat flour, baking soda, baking powder, cinnamon, and salt.
2. Mix in the milk, eggs, maple syrup, and melted butter.
3. Stir until everything is mixed.
4. Pour batter onto a greased griddle over medium heat.
5. Cook for about 2-3 minutes per side.
6. Serve it with pure maple syrup.

25. STEEL CUT OATS

Prep Time: 5 Mins

Cook Time: 25 Mins

Total Time: 30 Mins

Servings: 4

Ingredients

- 2 ½ cups of water plus additional as needed
- 1 cup of milk of any kind you like
- 1 cup of steel-cut oats
- ¼ tsp kosher salt do not omit this!

Instructions

1. In a medium or large saucepan, combine 2 ½ cups of water and milk. Over high heat, bring the water to a boil.
2. Mix in the oats and salt as soon as the liquid begins to boil. Bring it back to a steady boil., then immediately drop the heat to low, allowing the oats to simmer gently. At this point, don't leave the pot, because oats sometimes boil over. If your oats begin to froth and you are concerned, remove the pan from the heat and allow it to settle before returning it to the heat to finish cooking.
3. Allow the oats to slowly simmer for 20 minutes, stirring regularly and scraping the pan's bottom to prevent sticking. At this point, decide whether you want your oatmeal chewy or creamy. Continue cooking for 5 to 10 minutes more, stirring every few minutes, until the oatmeal is as soft as you want it. If the oatmeal becomes too dense, add a splash more water or milk to thin it out until it's the right consistency.
4. Remove the oats from the heat and set them aside for a few minutes to thicken. Serve it hot with your favorite toppings.

Notes

1. Leftover steel-cut oatmeal is a meal planner's dream! Refrigerate leftovers for up to 5 days, either in one huge batch or in individual portions. As it cools, the oatmeal will thicken. gradually reheat in the microwave or on the stove with an additional splash of liquid to thin it up.
2. Steel-cut oats are also great for freezing. Refrigerate for up to 3 months in an airtight container. Thaw in the fridge overnight.

26. CHEESY ZUCCHINI CASSEROLE

Prep Time: 10 Mins

Cook Time: 35 Mins

Total Time: 45 Mins

Servings: 6

Ingredients

- 2 medium zucchini, quartered and chopped
- 2 tbsp butter, cut into small pieces
- 3 large eggs
- ¼ cup of heavy cream
- ¼ cup of chopped onion
- ½ tsp salt
- ½ tsp pepper
- 6 ounces of divided shredded cheddar
- ¼ cup of grated Parmesan cheese
- ¼ cup of finely crushed pork rinds (or parmesan crisps)

Instructions

1. Bring to a boil a big pot of lightly salted water. Cook until the zucchini is just soft, approximately 4 minutes. In a colander, drain thoroughly.
2. Preheat the oven to 350 degrees Fahrenheit. Oil a 9-inch round or 8-inch square ceramic baking sheet with cooking spray. Spread the zucchini in the pan and dot with butter bits.
3. Mix together the eggs and cream in a large mixing bowl. Combine the onions, salt, pepper, and half of the cheddar cheese in a mixing bowl. Pour the sauce over the zucchini.
4. Sprinkle the remaining cheddar, parmesan, and pork rinds on top. Cook for 35 minutes, or until the top is bubbling and the edges are well browned. If desired, top with chopped basil.

27. EGGPLANT AND GOAT CHEESE SANDWICHES

Total Time: 40 Mins

Servings: 2

Ingredients

- 8 (½-inch-thick) eggplant slices
- 2 tsp divided olive oil
- 1 large red bell pepper
- 1-ounce ciabatta bread
- 2 tbsp of refrigerated pesto
- 1 cup of baby arugula
- ⅛ tsp freshly ground black pepper
- 2 ounces of soft goat cheese

Instructions

1. Preheat your broiler.
2. Put slices of eggplant in a single layer on a baking sheet that has been coated with foil. 1 tsp of oil on both sides of the eggplant. Cut the bell pepper in half lengthwise and remove the seeds and membrane. Place bell pepper halves, skin sides up, on a baking sheet with the eggplant; flatten with your hand. After 4 minutes of boiling, turn the eggplant over (do not turn the bell pepper over). Broil for 4 minutes more; remove eggplant from pan. Broil the bell pepper for another 7 minutes or until browned. Place the bell pepper in a zip-top plastic bag and seal it. Allow it sit for 15 minutes; then peel and discard the skin.
3. Broil bread slices for 2 minutes, rotating once, or until lightly browned. 1 tbsp of pesto on each of the 2 bread slices. Layer 2 eggplant slices, 1 bell pepper half, and 2 eggplant slices on each bread piece, pesto side up. Stir the arugula with the remaining 1 tsp of oil and black pepper, then divide it evenly between the sandwiches. Put 2 tbsp of goat cheese on each of the remaining bread pieces; arrange them, cheese side down, on sandwiches.

28. VEGAN BREAKFAST POTATO BOWL

Prep Time: 15 Mins

Cook Time: 30 Mins

Total Time: 45 Mins

Servings: 4

Ingredients

Potato hash

- 2 tsp of coconut oil (see directions for oil-free)
- 680g of chopped russet potatoes
- 160g diced white onion
- 180g diced tomato
- 75g diced red bell pepper
- salt and freshly ground black pepper
- 20g firmly packed arugula

Mushroom gravy

- 355ml plus 1 tbsp divided light coconut milk
- 80g diced white onion
- 2 minced garlic cloves
- 35g diced baby bella mushrooms
- 1 tbsp cornstarch
- 3 tbsp of nutritional yeast
- vegan cheese shreds, for topping (optional)
- 1 tbsp liquid aminos

Instructions

1. **Potato hash:** In a large saucepan, melt the coconut oil over medium-high heat. Put the potatoes in when the pan is heated enough to make the water sizzle. Cook, covered, for 15 minutes, stirring constantly. (If you can, start your gravy now.) NOTE: Instead of oil, I used broth and a nonstick pan.
2. Cover and sauté the onions in the potatoes until they are transparent. Reduce the heat and add the tomatoes and pepper. Cook until the potatoes are crispy and cooked all the way through, uncovered.

3. Sprinkle with salt to taste. Fold in the arugula just before serving so that it does not become too limp.
4. **Mushroom gravy:** If you can, make the gravy at the same time as the potatoes. I wouldn't recommend doing it after, because the potatoes might get mushy when reheated.
5. 1 tbsp of coconut milk coats a medium pot. Bring it to a low boil over medium heat. Next, add the onion, cook it for 2 minutes, and then stir in the garlic. Add the mushrooms once the onions are almost translucent. Sauté the mushrooms until they have darkened and shrunk in size.
6. Toss the onion-mushroom mixture with the cornstarch to coat evenly. Place the contents of the saucepan, together with the remaining coconut milk, nutritional yeast, and liquid aminos, in a blender or food processor and pulse a few times for a smoother texture.
7. Return the gravy to the pot and heat to a boil. Reduce the heat so the gravy simmers. Stir or whisk every few minutes until the required thickness is reached, then season with pepper.
8. Divide the potato hash into four bowls (don't forget to fold in the arugula first!) and top with the cheese shreds and gravy, if using. Serve right away.

29. ANTI INFLAMMATORY SMOOTHIE

Prep Time: 5 Mins

Blending Time: 2 Mins

Total Time: 7 Mins

Servings: 2

Ingredients

- 1 cup of kale
- ½ beet peeled and chopped
- ½ cup of water
- ½ peeled orange
- 1 cup of mixed berries frozen
- ½ cup of pineapple frozen
- 1 tsp ginger root grated or chopped
- 1 tsp coconut oil
- 1 serving Protein Smoothie Boost optional

Instructions

1. In a blender, combine the baby kale, beet, water, and orange.
2. Blend until smooth.
3. Combine the remaining ingredients.
4. Blend one more until smooth.

Notes

1. Beets may be replaced by carrots.
2. Mango may be substituted for pineapple.
3. To make the smoothie less bitter, use baby kale or spinach.

30. VANILLA BEAN PUDDING

Total Time: 20 Mins

Servings: 6

Ingredients

- 2 ½ cups of 2% reduced-fat milk
- 1 vanilla bean, split lengthwise
- ¾ cup of sugar
- 3 tbsp cornstarch
- ⅛ tsp salt
- ¼ cup of half-and-half
- 2 large egg yolks
- 4 tsp butter

Instructions

1. In a medium, heavy pot, heat the milk. Scrape the seeds from the vanilla bean and add them to the milk. Bring the water to a boil.
2. In a large bowl, mix cornstarch, sugar, and salt. Stir together half-and-half and egg yolks. Incorporate the egg yolk mixture into the sugar mixture. Gradually incorporate half of the warm milk into the sugar mixture while stirring continually. Return the boiling milk mixture to the pan and return to a boil. Cook for 1 minute, stirring continuously. Turn off the heat. Mix the butter in until it melts. Remove and discard the vanilla bean.

3. Pour the pudding into a bowl. Arrange the bowl in a large ice-filled bowl for 15 minutes, or until the pudding has cooled fully, stirring continuously. Wrap the surface of the pudding with plastic wrap and chill.
4. Omit the vanilla bean, salt, and butter; whisk in ¼ cup of reduced-fat creamy peanut butter once the custard has cooked.
5. Omit the vanilla bean for a coconut pudding variation. Replace ¾ cup of the milk with ¾ cup of light unsweetened coconut milk. Omit the butter and add ½ cup of toasted sweetened flakes coconut once the pudding has finished cooking.

31. GRILLED PEACHES WITH BERRY SAUCE

Total Time : 15 Mins

Servings: 4

Ingredients

- ½ of 10-ounce package of frozen raspberries in syrup, partially thawed
- 1- ½ tsp of lemon juice
- 2 medium peaches, peeled and halved
- 5 tsp brown sugar
- ¼ tsp ground cinnamon
- ½ tsp vanilla extract
- 1 tsp butter

Instructions

1. Puree raspberries and lemon juice in a blender or food processor until smooth. Remove and discard the seeds. Chill covered. Arrange the peach halves on a large piece of heavy-duty foil, cut side up (about 18 x 12 in.). Sprinkle brown sugar and cinnamon into the peach centers. Dot with butter and sprinkle with vanilla. Seal the foil around the peaches. Grill for 15 minutes over medium heat, or until well cooked. Spoon the raspberry sauce over the peaches to serve.

32. EASY RASPBERRY TARTS

Prep Time: 20 Mins

Cook Time: 35 Mins

Total Time: 55 Mins

Servings: 17

Ingredients

- 17 ready-made mini pie shells
- 2 cups of frozen raspberries
- Juice of half a lemon
- ½ cup of granulated sugar
- 3 tbsp of cornstarch

Instructions

2. Set the oven to 350°F and line a baking sheet with 12 mini pie shells. (If the pie shells are frozen, defrost them for about 15 minutes.)
3. In a large bowl, combine frozen raspberries and lemon juice. Then, sprinkle sugar and cornstarch over the raspberry mixture. Fill the small pies halfway with the mixture.
4. Bake until crust is golden, 20–25 minutes. Allow to cool on a rack.
5. Take one of your extra mini pie shells and roll it on a smooth surface until it is somewhat flat but keeps its size and form. Using a cookie cutter, cut out little hearts. Bake for 10 minutes on your baking sheet.
6. Place the cooked heart crusts in the center of the tarts and set aside to cool.

33. PUMPKIN PANCAKES

Prep Time: 10 Mins

Cook Time: 15 Mins

Total Time: 25 Mins

Servings: 6

Ingredients

- 1 ½ cups of milk
- 1 cup of pumpkin puree
- 1 large egg
- 2 tbsp of vegetable oil
- 2 tbsp of vinegar
- 2 cups of all-purpose flour
- 3 tbsp of brown sugar
- 2 tsp of baking powder
- 1 tsp baking soda
- 1 tsp ground allspice
- 1 tsp ground cinnamon
- ½ tsp ground ginger
- ½ tsp salt
- cooking spray

Instructions

1. Mix the egg, milk, pumpkin, oil, and vinegar in a large mixing bowl.
2. In an another bowl, combine the flour, brown sugar, baking powder, baking soda, allspice, cinnamon, ginger, and salt. Add it to the pumpkin mixture and stir until just mixed.
3. Cooking grease a griddle or frying pan and heat over medium-high heat.
4. Pour 3 to 4 tsp of batter onto the heated griddle for each pancake and flatten gently with a spoon. Cook for about 2 minutes, or until little bubbles emerge. Cook until golden brown on the other side, around 2 minutes more. Repeat with the remaining batter.

34. LEMON PARFAIT

Total Time: 15 Mins

Servings: 4

Ingredients

- 15 ounces of crumbled shortbread cookies
- 40 ounces of lemon pie filling
- 16 ounces of whipped topping

Instructions

1. Crumble 5 cookies into a glass (16-ounce stemless wine glass preferred), then add 14 cups of lemon pie filling on top, followed by 14 cup of whipped topping. Continue this process two additional times for a total of 3 layers.
2. Repeat step 1 in 3 additional glasses for a total of four full glasses.
3. You may serve it immediately or put it in the refrigerator until you're ready to serve it. Enjoy!

Notes

1. You do not need fine cookie crumbs because you are not preparing a pie crust. Just break the cookies into pieces that are about half an inch across.
2. The gorgeous layers set this dessert apart from others. Take your time to get clean layers.
3. Use wide, tall glasses to make them. If your glasses are narrow, it's definitely better to use a piping bag with the corner cut off to add the layers neatly.
4. You may add a layer of banana slices halfway down for a fruity twist. Mix the slices with lemon juice first, so they don't turn brown.

35. APPLE CINNAMON CRUMB MUFFINS

Prep Time: 25 Mins

Cook Time: 22 Mins

Total Time: 47 Mins

Servings: 14

Ingredients

- ⅓ cup of packed light sugar
- 1 tbsp granulated sugar
- 1 tsp ground cinnamon
- ¼ cup of melted unsalted butter
- ⅔ cup of all-purpose flour (spoon & leveled)

Muffins

- 1 and ¾ cups of all-purpose flour (spoon & leveled)
- 1 tsp baking soda
- 1 tsp baking powder
- 1 tsp ground cinnamon
- ½ tsp salt
- ½ cup of softened unsalted butter, to room temperature
- ½ cup of packed light or dark brown sugar
- ¼ cup of granulated sugar
- 2 large eggs, at room temperature
- ½ cup of yogurt or sour cream, at room temperature
- 2 tsp of pure vanilla extract
- ¼ cup of milk (any kind), at room temperature
- 1 and ½ cups of peeled & chopped apples (½ inch chunks)
- Vanilla icing (optional)
- 1 cup of confectioners' sugar
- 3 tbsp of heavy cream
- ½ tsp pure vanilla extract

Instructions

1. Preheat the oven to 425 degrees Fahrenheit. Spray or line a 12-count muffin tin with nonstick cooking spray. This recipe yields up to 14 muffins, so you may need a second pan, but you can always bake in batches with just one pan. Place aside.

2. **To make the crumbs:** In a medium mixing bowl, combine the brown sugar, granulated sugar, and cinnamon. With a fork, combine the melted butter and flour. Do not over-mix the mixture and keep it in big crumbles. Over-mixing will result in a thick paste. Set aside the topping.

3. **Make the muffins:** Combine the flour, baking soda, baking powder, cinnamon, and salt in a large mixing bowl and set aside.

4. Mix the sugar and butter on high for 2 minutes, or until smooth and creamy. As required, scrape down the sides and bottom of the bowl. Combine the eggs, yogurt, and vanilla essence in a bowl. 1 minute on medium speed and then 1 minute on high speed until the mixture is blended and mostly creamy. (It's fine if it seems curdled.) As required, scrape down the sides and bottom of the bowl. Add the dry ingredients and milk to the wet ingredients while the mixer is running on low speed, and beat until no flour pockets remain. Incorporate the apples.

5. Fill each cup or liner all the way to the top with the batter. Crumble topping on top of each, carefully pushing it down, so it sticks.

6. Bake for 5 minutes at 425°F, then lower the oven temperature to 350°F while the muffins are still in the oven. Cook for 15–18 minutes more, or until a toothpick inserted into the middle comes out clean. The overall baking time for these muffins is 20–23 minutes. The muffins should cool in the pan for five minutes before being moved to a wire rack to finish cooling.

7. **Make the icing:** Mix together all the frosting ingredients and sprinkle over warm or cooled muffins.

8. Iced or plain muffins keep fresh for a few days at room temperature or up to a week in the refrigerated.

36. BLUEBERRY MUFFIN BITES

Prep Time: 50 Mins

Cook Time: 4 Hrs (chilling time)

Total Time: 4 Hrs 50 Mins

Servings: 12

Ingredients

- ¼ cup of nut or seed butter
- ¼ cup of applesauce
- ¼ cup of maple syrup
- ⅔ cup of coconut flour
- ½ tsp salt
- 1 tsp vanilla extract
- 1 cup of fresh blueberries

Instructions

1. Set the oven to 375 degrees.
2. Bake the blueberries for 40 to 45 minutes on a tray with parchment paper.
3. Take it from the oven, let it cool for 10–15 minutes, then separate the parchment paper.
4. Nut or seed butter, applesauce, maple syrup, and vanilla extract are all combined in a bowl.
5. Combine the salt and coconut flour.
6. Fold in the blueberries.
7. roll into 12 balls.
8. Keep chilled until hard (3–4 hours).
9. Enjoy! Keep it in a refrigerator.

37. BANANA WALNUT CAKE RECIPE

Prep Time: 10 Mins

Cook Time: 25 Mins

Total Time: 35 Mins

Servings: 6

Ingredients

- 120g of all-purpose flour
- 1 tsp Baking Powder
- ½ tsp Baking Soda
- ¼ tsp cardamom powder
- ½ tsp cinnamon powder
- 50 g Butter
- ¾ cup of Brown Sugar
- 1 ripe banana
- ½ cup of milk
- 1 egg
- ½ cup of Walnuts

Instructions

1. Set the oven to 180 degrees Celsius.
2. Prepare a small loaf pan or muffin mould with a little oil.
3. Combine the butter and sugar in a bowl.
4. Mix well after adding the egg and the mashed banana.
5. Mix thoroughly after adding the flour, baking soda, baking powder, cinnamon, and cardamom powder.
6. Add the milk and carefully fold.
7. Add walnuts and carefully fold.
8. Place it in a baking tray, sprinkle walnuts on top, and bake for 25 minutes.
9. Take out and warm serve.

38. HANDY SAUSAGE BISCUITS

Prep Time: 25 Mins

Bake Time: 10 Mins

Total Time: 35 Mins

Servings: 2 Dozen

Ingredients

- ¾ pound of bulk pork sausage
- 2⅔ cups of all-purpose flour
- 2 tbsp of sugar
- 1-½ tsp baking powder
- ½ tsp baking soda
- ½ tsp salt
- ¼ cup of warm water (110° to 115°)
- ½ cup of shortening
- 1 package active dry yeast
- 1 cup of buttermilk
- Melted butter

Instructions

1. Sausages should not be pink when cooked in a skillet over medium heat; drain thoroughly and put aside. Mix the sugar, flour, baking powder, baking soda, and salt in a bowl. Once the mixture is crumbly, add the shortening. Stir in the sausage.
2. In a separate dish, dissolve the yeast in the water and let aside for 5 minutes. Add in the buttermilk. Mix dry ingredients just enough to moisten them.
3. Gently knead the dough 6 to 8 times on a lightly floured surface. With a 2 in. biscuit cutter, roll out to a ½ in. thickness. Place them on lightly greased baking pans.
4. Apply butter to the top. Cook at 450 °F for 10–12 minutes, or until golden brown. Serve hot.

39. SIMPLE NO BAKE FRUIT TART

Prep Time: 20 Mins

Cook Time: 10 Mins

Total Time: 30 Mins

Servings: 12

Ingredients

Crust

- 1 ½ cups of graham cracker crumbs
- ½ cup of sliced almonds
- 8 tbsp of butter melted

Filling

- 8 ounces of cream cheese
- 1 cup of powdered sugar
- 8 ounce container of Cool Whip
- 1 tsp almond extract

Fresh Fruit Topping

- ½ -¾ pound strawberries sliced
- 1 pint of fresh blueberries
- 1 pint of fresh raspberries

Instructions

Crust

1. First, combine all crust ingredients in a blender or food processor until fully mixed.
2. Firmly press into an 11-inch tart pan or 9x13-inch pan.
3. If you prefer a no-bake crust, chill it for one hour in the fridge. If baking, set the oven to 350°F and cook for 8–10 minutes, or until gently browned.

Filling

4. Using a mixer or an electric mixer, combine the cream cheese and powdered sugar until light and frothy.

5. Mix in the Cool Whip and almond extract until thoroughly mixed. Top with fresh fruit and spread evenly over prepared crust.
6. Let it to chill for at least an hour. Serve cut into slices.

40. BEST BROWNIES

Prep Time: 15 Mins

Cook Time: 30 Mins

Total Time: 45 Mins

Servings: 16

Ingredients

- ½ cup of butter
- 1 cup of white sugar
- 2 eggs
- 1 tsp vanilla extract
- ⅓ cup of unsweetened cocoa powder
- ½ cup of all-purpose flour
- ¼ tsp salt
- ¼ tsp baking powder

Frosting

- 3 tbsp of softened butter
- 3 tbsp unsweetened cocoa powder
- 1 tbsp honey
- 1 tsp vanilla extract
- 1 cup of confectioners' sugar

Instructions

1. Heat the oven to 350°F. Grease and flour an 8-inch square baking sheet.
2. Melt ½ cup of butter in a large pot. Take it from the heat and mix in the sugar, eggs, and 1 tsp vanilla extract. Combine ⅓ cup of cocoa, ½ cup of flour, salt, and baking powder in a mixing bowl. Pour the batter into the prepared pan.
3. Bake for 25 to 30 minutes in a preheated oven. Do not overcook.

4. Take the brownies from the oven and prepare the frosting. 1 cup of confectioners' sugar, 3 tbsp melted butter, 3 tbsp cocoa, honey, 1 tsp vanilla essence. Stir until completely smooth.

5. While the brownies are still warm, frost them.

41. BROWNIE KISSES

Prep Time: 10 Mins

Cook Time: 10 Mins

Total Time: 20 Mins

Servings: 48

Ingredients

- 1 cup of butter room temp
- 4 ounces chopped semisweet chocolate
- 2 cups of sugar
- 1½ cups of all-purpose flour
- ½ cup of unsweetened cocoa
- 4 large eggs room temp
- 1 tsp pure vanilla extract
- ¾ tsp salt
- ¾ cup of mini chocolate chips

Instructions

1. Stir 1 cup of butter and 4 ounces of chocolate for 1 minute in the microwave. Heat in 30-second intervals, stirring constantly, until melted.
2. Mix together the sugar, flour, cocoa, eggs, vanilla, and salt. Combine the chocolate mixture with the dry ingredients. Stir in the chocolate chips. Don't over-blend. Pour batter into prepared muffin tins.
3. Cook at 350°F for 10 minutes for micro muffins and 15 to 18 minutes for regular size muffins. Take the pan out of the oven and quickly press a chocolate bar into the center.

42. CREAMY PEACHES

Total Time: 10 Mins

Servings: 4

Ingredients

- 15 ounces of sliced peaches in extra-light syrup, drained
- 1½ cups of fat-free cottage cheese
- 4 ounces fat-free cream cheese, cubed
- Sugar substitute equivalent to 1 tbsp sugar

Instructions

1. Set aside 4 thinly sliced peach slices for garnish. In a food processor, combine the remaining peaches and cottage cheese. Cover and process until smooth. Cover and process until the cream cheese and sugar substitute are combined.
2. Spoon into 4 serving bowls. Finish with the saved peaches. Refrigerate until ready to serve.

43. HEALTHIER DARK CHOCOLATE CHUNK OATMEAL COOKIE BARS

Prep Time: 10 Mins

Cook Time: 20 Mins

Total Time: 30 Mins

Servings: 24

Ingredients

- 2 ½ cups of old-fashioned oats
- 1 cup of all-purpose flour
- ½ tsp kosher salt
- 1 cup of white whole wheat
- ½ - ¾ cup of light brown sugar, or more for a sweeter cookie
- ¼ -½ cup of granulated sugar, or more for a sweeter cookie
- 1 tsp baking soda

- 1 cup of melted coconut oil
- 2 large eggs
- 1 tbsp vanilla extract
- 1 ½ cups of dark chocolate chunks

Instructions

1. Preheat the oven to 350 degrees Fahrenheit. Butter or line a 9x13-inch baking tray with parchment paper.
2. Mix the oats, flour, whole wheat flour, brown sugar, granulated sugar, baking soda, salt, coconut oil, eggs, and vanilla in a big bowl or the bowl of a stand mixer. Mix until all the ingredients are combine, and the dough is wet. The dough will be dry and crumbly. Mix in the chocolate bits.
3. Arrange the dough on the prepared baking tray. It will seem crumbly. Bake the bars for 18-20 minutes, or until the sides are firm and the bars are brown. Season with flaky salt (if desired). Allow to cool, then cut into bars.

44. LAYERED FRESH FRUIT SALAD

Prep Time: 20 Mins

Cook Time: 10 Mins + Cooling

Total Time: 30 Mins

Servings: 12

Ingredients

- ½ tsp grated orange zest
- ⅔ cup of orange juice
- ½ tsp grated lemon zest
- ⅓ cup of lemon juice
- ⅓ cup of packed light brown sugar
- 1 cinnamon stick

Fruit salad

- 2 cups of cubed fresh pineapple
- 2 cups of sliced fresh strawberries
- 2 medium kiwifruit, peeled and sliced

- 3 medium sliced bananas
- 2 medium oranges, peeled and sectioned
- 1 medium red grapefruit, peeled and sectioned
- 1 cup of seedless red grapes

Instructions

1. In a pan, boil the first 6 ingredients. Lower the heat to low and cook for 5 minutes, uncovered. Allow it to cool fully. Take out the cinnamon stick.
2. In a big glass bowl, layer the fruits. Pour the juice mixture on top. Refrigerate for several hours, covered.

45. NUTELLA HAZELNUT CHOCOLATE TRUFFLES

Total Time: 3 Hrs 20 Mins

Servings: 16

Ingredients

- 200g of high-quality dark chocolate, split up
- 120ml thickened or heavy cream
- 300g Nutella
- 120g skinless hazelnuts

Instructions

1. Place the dark chocolate in a small bowl and finely chop it. Next, heat the cream over the stove or in the microwave. After the cream has reached room temperature, pour it over the dark chocolate and put it aside for two minutes.
2. Stir the chocolate mixture slowly until it becomes a beautiful chocolate ganache. Continue mixing after adding half of the Nutella, then the remaining Nutella until mixed and smooth.
3. Arrange the chocolate in a small deep bowl and refrigerate for 2-3 hours, or until set.
4. Crush the hazelnuts until they are fine crumbs. Then, 1 heaping tsp at a time, scoop tbsp of the chocolate truffle mixture into your palms and roll them around until smooth, then roll them in the crushed hazelnuts. Keep truffles in the fridge.

Notes

1. Hazelnuts: Use either raw or roasted hazelnuts. To toast hazelnuts, place them in a small skillet over medium heat and shake until they turn brown and smell toasted. Remove from heat and cool.

46. RASPBERRY QUARK BAKED OATMEAL

Prep Time: 15 Mins

Cook Time: 40 Mins

Total Time: 55 Mins

Servings: 2

Ingredients

Main Batter

- 45g whole rolled oats lightly ground
- 250g raspberry wünder quark
- 1 egg separated
- 1 pinch of salt

Add-Ins

- 65g of frozen raspberries
- 25g sliced almonds

Instructions

Making the Batter

1. Preheat the oven to 350 degrees Fahrenheit.
2. Grind rolled oats to the consistency of fast oats in a blender or food processor.
3. Combine the oats, quark, and egg yolk in a large bowl.
4. Mix together the egg whites and salt until stiff peaks form. Fold the stiff egg white carefully into the quark, oat, and egg mixture, taking care not to deflate the egg white.

Assembling

5. Grease your baking sheet of choice. Place just half of the batter in the dish, then top with raspberries and the remaining batter.
6. Finally, sprinkle the sliced almonds on top of the batter.

Baking

7. Bake for 40 minutes—the baking time will vary a little depending on the size of your baking sheet. It should be plump and golden brown.
8. As it cools, the bake will collapse, but it still has a great flavor. I prefer to eat it right immediately, but it can be refrigerated for up to three days and reheated in the microwave.
9. I like to serve it with a bit of extra quark and some fresh raspberries!

Notes

1. This may be refrigerated for 3 days and reheated for a simple breakfast!

47. BEST HEALTHY CARROT MUFFINS WITH APPLESAUCE

Prep Time: 7 Mins

Cook Time: 25 Mins

Total Time: 32 Mins

Servings: 12

Ingredients

- 2 large eggs
- ¾ cup of unsweetened applesauce
- ⅓ cup of maple syrup or honey
- 1 tsp pure vanilla extract
- 1 tsp cinnamon
- ¾ tsp baking soda
- ½ tsp nutmeg
- 2 tsp baking powder
- ½ tsp salt
- 1 ½ cups of grated carrots packed

- 1 cup of whole wheat or spelt flour
- 1 cup of oat bran
- ⅓ cup of raisins or chopped dates, not packed
- ⅓ cup of coarsely chopped nuts (walnuts, pecans, hazelnuts)
- Cooking spray

Instructions

1. Set the oven to 350°F and coat a 12-muffin pan with nonstick cooking spray. Place aside.
2. Beat the eggs for 15 seconds in a large mixing bowl. Mix in the applesauce, maple syrup, vanilla, cinnamon, nutmeg, baking powder, baking soda, and salt.
3. Stir in the vegetables a few times. Mix in the oat bran or oats and whole wheat flour until well combined. Do not overmix. Mix in the raisins and nuts.
4. To bake, place a toothpick in the middle and bake for 25 minutes, or until the toothpick comes out clean, after dividing the batter evenly among the 12 openings of a pan. Take a few minutes for the muffins to cool before moving them to a cooling rack to cool completely.
5. In an airtight glass jar, keep in the refrigerator for up to a week. Freeze: Up to 3 months in an airtight container. You may defrost it in the refrigerator overnight or leave it out on the counter for 3 to 4 hours.

Notes

1. Muffins will rise less and be more substantial and chewy. Please don't confuse it with steel-cut oats, though.
2. **Yogurt:** Instead of applesauce, use plain standard or Greek yogurt.
3. **Jumbo or mini muffins:** You can make bigger or smaller muffins, but the baking time will need to be changed accordingly. Always do the toothpick test.
4. Baking is a science, and gluten-free flours such as almond flour or coconut flour will not bake as well as regular flour, so I do not suggest this substitution.
5. You can't use liquid stevia because it will change the amount of dry to wet ingredients, which will make the muffins fail. The same may be said for any dry sweetener.

48. MINI FRUIT TARTS

Prep Time: 30 Mins

Cook Time: 25 Mins

Tart Shell Freezing: 1 Hr

Total Time: 1 Hr 55 Mins

Servings: 6 mini tarts

Ingredients

Dough

- 1 ½ cups & 1 tbsp all-purpose flour
- ½ tsp salt
- 1 tbsp & 1 tsp powdered sugar
- 8 tbsp unsalted butter, cut into cubes
- 2 egg yolks
- ½ tsp vanilla extract
- 1 tbsp heavy cream

Custard filling

- 4 egg yolks
- 5 ½ tbsp white sugar
- 2 tbsp and 2 tsp all-purpose flour
- 2 tbsp and 2 tsp cornstarch
- 13.28 ounces of whole milk
- 1 tsp vanilla extract

Assembly

- Assorted sliced fresh fruits are
- 2 tbsp apricot jelly
- 1 ½ tbsp water

Instructions

Dough

1. Mix the flour, salt, sugar, and butter in a stand mixer fitted with the paddle attachment. Mix for one minute on the lowest level or until the butter is broken into tiny bits. Add each egg yolk, then add the heavy cream and vanilla essence.
2. Mix for about two minutes on medium (setting 4 or 6) or until the mixture like crumbly sand. Stop the mixer and squeeze some sandy dough between your fingers. You're ready to knead it if it sticks together and forms a ball. Add one spoonful of heavy cream at a time to correct the mixture's dryness.
3. Take the mixing bowl from the stand mixer and shape the sand into a ball of dough with your hand. I prefer to do this in a bowl because it makes less of a mess.
4. Scoop about three tsp of dough and form and flatten it straight into the tart molds with your hands. (For a four-inch tart shape, three tbsp equals approximately 60 grams of dough.)
5. Prick the bottom of each tart mold with a fork.
6. Chill the tarts in the molds for at least one hour before baking to prevent the dough from melting or shrinking in the oven.
7. Preheat the oven to 375 degrees Fahrenheit.
8. Bake your tarts in the oven for 12–15 minutes from the freezer. After about 8 minutes, check to see whether the centers of your tarts are rising. If they are rising, open the oven door and use a measuring cup to flatten the centers with light pressure. Continue to bake them until the edges start to brown, then remove them from the oven.
9. Take the tart shells out of the molds and allow them to cool on a rack. The finished shells should be a little hard to the touch. If you push the cores and they feel mushy or flex when you hold them up, they should be returned to their molds to finish baking for a few more minutes (make sure to keep an eye on these as they cook).
10. These tart shells may be made a few days before assembly; simply refrigerate them after they have cooled.

49. BUTTERY COCONUT BARS

Prep Time: 20 Mins

Bake Time: 40 Mins

Total Time: 1 Hr

Servings: 3

Ingredients

- 2 cups of all-purpose flour
- 1 cup of packed brown sugar
- ½ tsp salt
- 1 cup of melted butter

Filling

- 3 large eggs
- 14 ounces of sweetened condensed milk
- ½ cup of all-purpose flour
- ¼ cup of packed brown sugar
- ¼ cup of melted butter
- 3 tsp of vanilla extract
- ½ tsp salt
- 4 cups of sweetened shredded coconut

Instructions

1. Preheat the oven to 350 degrees. Line a 13x9-inch baking tray with parchment paper, letting the ends to reach up the edges.
2. Mix flour, brown sugar, and salt in a large bowl; stir in 1 cup of melted butter. Press into the prepared pan's bottom. 12–15 minutes until light brown. Allow to cool for 10 minutes on a wire rack. Reduce the oven temperature to 325°.
3. Stir together the first 7 filling ingredients in a large bowl. Add the coconut and mix well. Pour over crust and top with the remaining coconut. Cook for 25–30 minutes, or until light golden brown. Cool in the pan using a wire rack. Remove from pan using parchment paper. Cut the bars.

50. MARSHMALLOW BROWNIES

Prep Time: 30 Mins

Cook Time: 30 Mins

Total Time: 1 Hr

Servings 24

Ingredients

For the Brownie Base

- 4 ounces of unsweetened chocolate
- ⅔ cup of unsalted butter
- 1¼ cups of semisweet chocolate chips, divided
- 1⅓ cups of all-purpose flour
- 1 tsp baking powder
- ½ tsp salt
- 4 eggs at room temperature
- 2 cups of granulated sugar
- 2 tsp of vanilla extract

For the Marshmallow Layer

- 10.5 ounce bag miniature marshmallows

For the Crispy Chocolate Peanut Butter Layer

- 1½ cups of milk chocolate chips
- 1 cup of smooth peanut butter
- 1 tbsp unsalted butter
- 1½ cups of Rice Krispies cereal

Instructions

1. Prepare the cookies: Set the oven temperature to 350° Fahrenheit. Grease a 9x13-inch baking pan.
2. Melt the unsweetened chocolate, butter, and 3/4 cup of semisweet chocolate chips in a medium saucepan over medium heat. While melting, stir occasionally. Set aside for 5 minutes to cool.

3. Mix the eggs well in a large bowl. Add the sugar and vanilla extract and mix until everything is well mixed. Mix the melted components into the egg mixture well. After sifting them, mix the flour, baking powder, and salt well together. Incorporate the remaining ½ cup of semisweet chocolate chips.
4. Smooth the batter into an equal layer in the prepared pan. Cook for 25-30 minutes, or until a wooden skewer into the pan comes out wet with crumbs.
5. Take the brownies from the oven and immediately top with the marshmallows. Return the pan to the oven for 3 minutes longer.
6. Prepare the Crispy Chocolate Peanut Butter Layer: Meanwhile, in a medium saucepan, combine the milk chocolate chips, peanut butter, and 1 tbsp of butter. Melt over low heat, continually stirring, until fully melted. Take it from the heat and stir in the rice treats. Allow three minutes for cooling.
7. Evenly distribute the mixture over the marshmallow layer. Let it cool to room temperature before refrigerating for 30 minutes to make slicing easier. The brownies may be kept at room temperature or in the fridge for up to one week.

Notes

1. Equipment: 9x13-inch baking pan
2. Brownies: Make a 9x13-inch pan of brownies using your favorite brownie recipe (or a box mix!).
3. Note on Peanut Butter: Natural peanut butter is too oily to use.
4. Substitutes for peanut butter: I've successfully made the top layer with Sunbutter (Natural Sunbutter with the yellow lid) and almond butter (Barney Butter smooth).
5. Storage: Keep the brownies in an airtight container at room temperature or in the fridge for up to 1 week.
6. Wrap each brownies in plastic wrap and freeze for up to 3 months in an airtight container or freezer bag. Allow to thaw at room temperature.

51. MINI RASPBERRY TARTS

Prep Time: 20 Mins

Cook Time: 11 Mins

Total Time: 31 Mins

Servings : 32

Ingredients

- 16.5-ounce refrigerated sugar cookie dough
- 8-ounce ⅓-less fat block-style cream cheese
- ¼ cup of sugar
- 1 orange Zest
- ½ tsp vanilla extract
- 32 fresh raspberries

Instructions

1. Preheat the oven to 350 degrees. nonstick cooking spray a mini-muffin tin. Make 32 pieces of sugar cookie dough. Dust some flour on your hands and roll each of the pieces into a ball. Press each ball into the tin, forming the dough into the shape of a tart. Bake for 11–12 minutes, or until brown. Cooling for ten minutes in the pan. Cool the tarts thoroughly on a cooling rack. Mix cream cheese, sugar, orange zest, and vanilla extract in an electric mixer. Put the cream cheese mixture into each tart. Finish with a fresh raspberry on top of each. Refrigerate until ready to serve.

52. PEANUT BUTTER STUFFED APPLES

Prep Time: 5 Mins

Cook Time: 30 Mins

Total Time: 35 Mins

Servings : 6

Ingredients

- 3 apples, halved
- 2 tbsp melted butter
- 1 cup of creamy peanut butter
- ¼ cup of chopped Reese's Pieces
- ⅔ cup of melted semisweet chocolate chips

Instructions

2. Preheat the oven to 375 degrees. Core the apples with a melon baller. Brush the apples with melted butter in a shallow baking sheet. Bake for 15 minutes.
3. Take the apples from the oven and fill each with a large scoop of peanut butter. Bake for an additional 15 minutes. Decorate with Reese's Pieces and melted chocolate drizzle.

53. GRILLED PEACHES WITH BERRY SAUCE

Total Time: 15 Mins

Grill Time: 15 Mins

Total Time: 30 Mins

Servings : 4

Ingredients

- ½ of 10-ounce package of frozen raspberries in syrup, partially thawed
- 1-½ tsp of lemon juice
- 2 medium peaches, peeled and halved
- 5 tsp brown sugar
- ¼ tsp ground cinnamon
- ½ tsp vanilla extract
- 1 tsp butter

Instructions

1. Puree raspberries and lemon juice in a blender or food processor until smooth. Remove and discard the seeds. Cover and cool down. Arrange the peach halves on a large piece of heavy-duty foil, cut side up (about 18 x 12 in.). Pour brown sugar and cinnamon into the peach centers. Dot with butter and sprinkle with vanilla. Seal the foil around the peaches. Grill for 15 minutes over medium heat, or until well cooked. Spoon the raspberry sauce over the peaches to serve.

54. QUICK APPLE CRISP

Total Time: 30 Mins

Servings: 8

Ingredients

- 1 cup of graham cracker crumbs
- ½ cup of all-purpose flour
- ½ cup of packed brown sugar
- 1 tsp ground cinnamon
- ½ tsp ground nutmeg
- ½ cup of melted butter
- 8 medium tart apples, peeled and sliced
- whipped topping or ice cream

Instructions

2. Mix the cracker crumbs, flour, brown sugar, cinnamon, nutmeg, and butter in a large bowl. Place the apples in a greased 2- ½ -quart microwave-safe dish. Crumble mixture on top.
3. Microwave for 8–9 minutes, uncovered, on high, or until apples are soft. Serve it hot with whipped cream or ice cream.

55. BEST CHOCOLATE CHIP COOKIES

Prep Time: 20 Mins

Cook Time: 10 Mins

Additional: 30 Mins

Total Time: 1 Hr

Servings: 24

Ingredients

- 1 cup of softened butter
- 1 cup of white sugar
- 1 cup of packed brown sugar
- 2 eggs
- 2 tsp of vanilla extract
- 1 tsp baking soda
- 2 tsp of hot water
- ½ tsp salt
- 3 cups of all-purpose flour
- 2 cups of semisweet chocolate chips
- 1 cup of chopped walnuts

Instructions

1. Preheat the oven to 350°F.
2. Cream the white sugar, butter, and brown sugar together until smooth. One at a time, combine the eggs, and then the vanilla extract. Dissolve baking soda in boiling water. Combine it with the salt in the batter. Mix in the flour, chocolate chips, and nuts. Using a big spoon, drop them into ungreased pans.
3. In a preheated oven, cook for around 10 minutes or until the sides are thoroughly browned.

56. CHOCOLATE CHUNK COOKIES WITH SEA SALT

Prep Time: 1 Hr

Cook Time: 16 Mins

Total Time: 1 Hr 16 Mins

Servings: 16

Ingredients

- ¼ cup of softened unsalted butter, to room temperature
- ½ cup of light brown sugar, packed
- 2 tbsp granulated sugar
- 1 ½ tsp vanilla extract
- 1 large egg, room temperature
- 1 ¼ cups of all-purpose flour
- ½ tsp baking soda
- ½ tsp baking powder
- ¼ tsp flaky sea salt and more salt for topping
- 1 cup of chocolate chunks (plus more if needed)

Instructions

1. Heat the oven to 350°F.
2. If using a stand mixer or a mixing bowl and spoon, combine the butter and both sugars. To dissolve the sugar in the butter, mix for approximately 2 minutes. Mix in the vanilla and egg until well combined, scraping down the sides of the bowl as necessary.
3. Just mix the flour, baking soda, and baking powder by sifting them all together and stirring briefly. Add the chocolate pieces and stir them in with a spatula. Place it in the fridge for 30 minutes or in the freezer for 15 minutes. This lets the butter firm up and keeps the cookies from spreading too much.
4. Scoop 2 tsp of dough and place them 3 inches (8 cm) apart on a cookie sheet. If you really want to be sure they're all the same size, weigh them each to 1.2 ounces (34 grams). Use your palm to slightly smooth the top and add extra pieces if required.
5. If your baking pan is darker, reduce the baking time to 16 to 18 minutes. The sides should be golden brown in color. Take it from the oven and immediately sprinkle with flaky sea salt.

6. Allow the cookies to cool for a few minutes on the pan. Put it on a cooling rack to cool fully. They may be kept at room temperature in a sealed container for up to 4 days.

57. CHOCOLATE COVERED STRAWBERRY CUBES

Total Time: 4 Hs 10 Mins

Servings: 16

Ingredients

- 2 cups of chocolate chips
- 2 tbsp coconut oil
- 16 fresh strawberries with stems

Instructions

1. In a medium mixing bowl, combine melted chocolate chips and coconut oil.
2. Fill each ice cube form with a coating of chocolate mixture, then top with a strawberry, stem side up. Distribute the remaining chocolate mixture over the strawberries.
3. Freeze for 4 to 5 hours, or until the chocolate is firm.

58. EASY CINNAMON SAUTÉED PEARS

Prep Time: 5 Mins

Cook Time: 10 Mins

Total Time: 15 Mins

Servings: 4

Ingredients

- 2 large pears
- 2 tsp oil
- 2 tbsp water
- 1 tsp ground cinnamon

Instructions

1. Peel, core, and slice pears into ½ -inch thick slices.
2. In a pan, heat the oil over medium-low heat.
3. Pour in the pears, water, and cinnamon. Stir.
4. Simmer, occasionally stirring, until the pears are cooked and caramelized, around 10-15 minutes.

Notes

1. Refrigerate leftovers in an airtight jar for up to 4 days.
2. Leave the peel on if you want more fiber and less prep labor.

59. WHITE CHOCOLATE COOKIES

Prep Time: 10 Mins

Cook Time: 12 Mins

Total Time: 22 Mins

Servings: 10

Ingredients

-   120 g of softened unsalted butter
-   85 g light brown soft sugar
-   65 g golden caster sugar
-   1 medium egg
-   1 tsp vanilla bean paste
-   180 g plain flour
-   ½ tsp of bicarbonate of soda
-   180g white chocolate, broken into chunks

Instructions

1. Set the oven to 180 degrees Celsius (160 degrees Celsius fan/gas 4) and line two big baking sheets with parchment paper. Mix the sugar and butter in a big bowl using an electric mixer or a stand mixer until just incorporated. Crack in the egg and continue to beat. Mix in the vanilla, flour, bicarb, chocolate pieces, and ¼ tsp of fine sea salt.

2. Roll the ingredients into 10 even-sized balls between your palms. Cook for 10–12 minutes, or until brown around the sides, on prepared baking trays. Transfer it to a cooling rack and allow it to cool fully, or serve it warm with ice cream.

60. BLACKBERRY CRUMBLE

Prep Time: 10 Mins

Cook Time 40 Mins

Total Time 50 Mins

Servings: 8

Ingredients

Fruit Filling

- 6 cups of fresh blackberries
- ⅓ cup of all-purpose flour
- ⅓ cup of granulated sugar

Crumble Topping:

- ⅔ cup of old-fashioned oats
- ½ cup of dark brown sugar
- ¼ cup of all-purpose flour
- 3 tbsp softened butter
- 1 tbsp vegetable oil
- 1 tsp ground cinnamon
- ¼ tsp table salt

Instructions

1. Preheat the oven to 375 °F.
2. Mix blackberries, sugar, and all-purpose flour in a large bowl. Place on an 8 x 8 baking sheet.
3. For the crumble topping, place all of the ingredients in a medium mixing bowl and mix with hands until the mixture resembles a crumble.
4. Crumble the topping over the blackberry mixture. Cook the crumble for 40 minutes, or until the topping is golden brown and the blackberries are bubbling. Allow for a

15-minute cooling period before serving. If preferred, serve it warm or at room temperature with ice cream.

61. FLATBREAD PIZZA

Prep Time: 15 Mins

Cook Time: 35 Mins

Total Time: 50 Mins

Servings: 3

Ingredients

For flatbread

- 2 cups of all-purpose flour, extra for the surface
- 2 tsp baking powder
- 1 tsp kosher salt
- ½ tsp baking soda
- 1 cup of plain Greek yogurt
- 2 tbsp olive oil
- Vegetable oil for the pan

For topping

- 12-ounce grape tomatoes, halved
- ¼ small sliced red onion
- 2 tsp extra-virgin olive oil
- 2 tsp freshly chopped oregano
- Kosher salt
- freshly ground black pepper
- 8 ounces of mozzarella, sliced into ¼" thick rounds
- Balsamic glaze, for serving
- 2 cups of arugula

Instructions

1. Preheat the oven to 400 degrees. Mix the flour, baking soda, salt, and baking powder in a large bowl. Stir in the yogurt and oil until no dry areas remain.

2. Flour a clean work surface lightly. Move the dough to a worktop and knead it for three to four minutes, or until the dough is smooth. Add a bit of more flour if the dough is too sticky.

3. Roll each dough piece to ¼" thickness. Warm enough vegetable oil to cover the bottom of a big pan or griddle over medium-high heat. Cook flatbreads for 2 minutes or until brown on both sides. Cook the flatbreads further, using extra vegetable oil as necessary. Mix tomatoes, red onion, oil, and oregano in a medium bowl and season with salt and pepper. Top each flatbread with the tomato-onion mixture and bake for 15 minutes, or until the cheese is melted. Arugula and balsamic glaze should be drizzled on top before serving.

62. BLUEBERRY PEACH COBBLER

Prep Time: 20 Mins

Cook Time: 50 Mins

Total Time: 1 Hr 10 Mins

Servings: 9

Ingredients

- 1 ½ cups of sliced fresh or frozen peaches
- 1 cup of fresh or frozen blueberries
- ¼ cup of granulated sugar
- 8 tbsp of unsalted butter
- 1 cup of all-purpose flour
- 1 cup of granulated sugar
- ½ cup of whole milk
- 1 ½ tsp baking powder
- ½ tsp salt

Instructions

1. If using fresh fruit, gently combine the peaches, blueberries, and ¼ cup of sugar in a bowl and set aside for 30 minutes, stirring occasionally.

2. If you're using frozen fruit, in a large bowl, mix the peaches and berries and set aside for 20–30 minutes, or until the fruit has partially thawed. If the fruit has generated a lot of juice, drain it and place it back in the bowl. Add ¼ cup of sugar

and set alone for another 10 to 20 minutes to allow the sugar to dissolve. (The fruit will release more liquid, but you don't want to drain it yet.)

3. Set the oven to 350°F once the mixture has sat for 30 minutes.
4. Melt the butter in the bottom of an 11-by-7-inch (or 9-inch-square) baking sheet.
5. In a bowl, combine the flour, remaining 1 cup of sugar, milk, baking powder, and salt until combined. Pour the melted butter over the top.
6. Pour the fruit (and all of its juices) over the batter. There will appear to be a lot of liquid, but this is typical. Avoid stirring or swirling the batter and the fruit together!
7. Place the baking sheet on a wide baking sheet to catch any spilled liquids, and bake for 48 to 58 minutes, or until the fruit has sunken to the bottom of the skillet and the top of the cobbler is golden brown.
8. Let it to cool for 30 minutes to an hour—longer is fine—to allow the juices to set before serving with ice cream, whipped cream, or even just a dusting of powdered sugar. However, ice cream is highly recommended!
9. Uneaten cobbler can be refrigerated for up to 3 days, covered. (Be sure to totally cool your cobbler before covering and refrigerating it, or it will sweat.)
10. Slices of cobbler can also be frozen in sealed containers for approximately a month. Thaw in the microwave or the refrigerator overnight.

Notes

1. If you use fresh peaches, you'll need 2 to 3 (depending on size).
2. If your fruit isn't extremely sweet, you can add up to ¼ cup of more sugar. If desired, you can reduce the amount of sugar added to the fruit. (Adjust only the amount of sugar mixed in with the fruit, not the amount in the cobbler topping.)

63. GOLDEN TURMERIC ENERGY BALLS

Prep Time: 5 Mins

Cook Time: 5 Mins

Total Time: 10 Mins

Servings: 25

Ingredients

- 1 cup of almonds, raw
- 1 cup of walnuts raw
- ½ cup of dried cranberries
- 1 cup of shredded coconut
- 1 tbsp turmeric powder
- ⅛ tsp salt
- ⅛ tsp black pepper
- 5 dates medjool

Instructions

1. Begin by blitzing the nuts in a blender or food processor until they are little pieces. They don't have to become too powdery because the thicker texture is preferable for your energy balls.
2. Next, add the rest of the items and mix them well. Make sure the dates and cranberries are thoroughly mixed into the mixture.
3. Spoon out a little of the mixture and attempt to roll it into a ball. If it stays, fantastic; if the ball breaks apart easily, add another Medjool date and combine again. You could also add 1 tbsp of coconut oil.
4. Roll the mixture into balls after it has become sufficiently sticky. You may use gloves to prevent your hands from being stained since turmeric will stain everything.
5. These energy balls may then be refrigerated for 5 days or frozen for up to 6 months in an airtight container.

Notes

1. If your dates are a touch dry, soak them for 10 minutes in hot water before adding them to the mixer. This way, you won't have to add more dates or coconut oil to the recipe for energy balls.
2. Recipe Variations for Energy Balls:

3. You could make a few substitutions for this recipe. Obviously, each change will change how the final no-bake energy balls taste overall. It does, however, allow for some experiment. As an example:
4. Other nuts may replace almonds and walnuts, such as pistachios or your personal favorites. Almond butter and nut butters are used in some energy ball recipes to help generate a sticky mixture. However, I prefer chunks of raw nuts in mine.
5. Dried cranberries help with stickiness and flavor. However, other dried fruit, such as apricot or peaches, might be used.
6. You can also use other soft dried fruits like apricots instead of Medjool dates. They provide sweetness and help bind the recipe. Different elements influence the outcome.
7. For a higher protein snack, add some flax seeds or chia seeds (or even protein powder) to the mix.
8. Feel free to flavor them further with homemade vanilla essence or raw cacao powder.
9. To make the turmeric energy balls even sweeter, feel free to sprinkle the mixture with maple syrup. Just be careful not to over-wet it.
10. Add some chocolate chips for a more dessert-like snack. They actually taste fantastic with the almonds, coconut, and dates.

64. SOUR VINEGAR AND CHILI OIL SAUCE

Prep Time: 25 Mins

Cook Time: 1 Hr 25 Mins

Total Time: 1 Hr 50 Mins

Serves:8

Ingredients

for the wontons

- 454g of ground pork shoulder
- 6g kosher salt
- 13g sugar
- 2g finely ground white pepper
- 1 ½ ounces minced scallions or Chinese chives
- 2 tsp minced fresh garlic

- 40 thin, square wonton wrappers
- 10ml Shaoxing wine or dry sherry

For the sauce:

- 4–8 whole hot Chinese dried red peppers, stems removed
- ¼ cup of vegetable or canola oil
- 2 tsp of Sichuan peppercorns
- 1 tbsp of roasted sesame oil
- 1 tbsp toasted sesame seeds
- 3 tbsp Chinkiang vinegar
- 1 tbsp sugar
- 1 tbsp minced fresh garlic
- 2 tbsp soy sauce

To Cook and Serve:

- 2 tbsp of minced fresh cilantro leaves and fine stems
- 2 tbsp of lightly crushed roasted peanuts (optional)

Instructions

1. In a medium bowl, knead and turn the pork, salt, sugar, white pepper, scallions, garlic, and wine until the mixture is homogenous and begins to feel tacky/sticky around 1 minute. Transfer a tsp-sized quantity to a microwave-safe plate and microwave on high power for 10 seconds or until cooked through. Sprinkle with more salt, white pepper, or sugar to taste.
2. Set up a workstation with a small bucket of water, a clean dish towel for wiping your fingers, a bowl of wonton filling, a parchment-lined rimmed baking sheet for the finished wontons, and a stack of wrapped wonton wrappers.
3. To make dumplings, place one wrapper on top of a flat hand. Put a 2 tsp- to 1 tbsp-sized quantity of filling in the center of the wrapper with a spoon. Use the tip of your other hand's finger to lightly wet the wrapper's edge with water (do not use too much water). Wipe your fingers dry with a kitchen towel.
4. Fold one wonton wrapper tip across to meet the opposite tip to make a triangle. Seal the triangle's edges, carefully squeezing out all air from within the wrapping as you do. Bring the two hypotenuse corners of the freshly created triangle together, moistening one with a bit of water, crossing them, and pinching to seal. Place the completed dumplings on a baking sheet lined with parchment paper.

5. To make the sauce: Microwave the chilies and Sichuan peppercorns on high for about 15 seconds, or until toasted and fragrant. Smashed in a mortar and pestle or food processor to resemble crushed red pepper flakes. Place it in a small saucepan.

6. Add the oil to a pan and bring it to a boil over medium-high heat. Pour heated oil over the chile/peppercorn mixture right away (it should sizzle). Transfer it after 5 minutes of cooling to a medium bowl. Set aside the sesame oil.

7. In a bowl, mix together the vinegar, sugar, soy sauce, and garlic until the sugar dissolves. Pour in the chili oil mixture. Save until ready to use. (Sealed sauce may be refrigerated for 2 weeks.)

8. **To prepare and serve:** Bring a big saucepan of water to a boil. Cook until 12 to 16 wontons are thoroughly cooked through, around 4 minutes. Transfer wontons to a heated serving plate. Pour the sauce over the top. Serve immediately with peanuts and cilantro chopped.

65. ZUCCHINI MUFFINS

Prep Time: 15 Mins

Cook Time: 25 Mins

Total Time: 40 Mins

Servings: 12

Ingredients

- 2 large eggs
- 270g sugar
- 2 tsp of vanilla extract
- 3 cups of packed grated zucchini
- ¾ cup of melted unsalted butter
- 2 ¾ cups of all-purpose flour
- 1 tsp baking soda
- 1 tsp baking powder
- ¼ tsp salt
- 2 tsp of cinnamon
- 1 tsp ground ginger
- ½ tsp nutmeg
- 1 cup of walnuts, optional
- 1 cup of raisins or dried cranberries, optional

Instructions

1. Preheat the oven to 350 degrees Fahrenheit.
2. Prepare the batter
3. Beat the eggs in a large bowl. Mix the sugar and vanilla essence in a bowl. Combine the grated zucchini and the melted butter in a bowl. Mix the flour, cinnamon, baking powder, baking soda, powdered ginger, nutmeg, and salt in a separate bowl.
4. To make the batter:
5. Combine the dry ingredients with the zucchini mixture. (Do not over-mix!) If using, mix with walnuts, raisins, or cranberries.
6. Fill muffin cups with fill.
7. Brush a little butter or vegetable oil spray into each muffin cup in your muffin pan. Using a spoon, divide the muffin dough evenly among the muffin cups, filling the muffin tin all the way to the top.
8. Now cook the muffins in the middle of the oven at 350 degrees Fahrenheit for 20-30 minutes, till the tops are lightly browned and spring back when pressed. Use a long toothpick or a thin bamboo stick to ensure that the muffins' centers are done.

66. BANANA SMOOTHIE

Total Time: 5 Mins

Servings: 1

Ingredients

1. 1 cup of sliced banana, frozen is best
2. ¼ cup of Greek yogurt, plain or vanilla
3. ¼ cup of milk, dairy, almond, oat milk, etc.
4. ¼ tsp vanilla extract

Instructions

1. Put all of the ingredients in a mixer and blend them together. Blend until smooth, adding additional milk to get the desired consistency.
2. Serve right away.

Notes

1. Frozen banana thickens and freezes the smoothie. If your banana is not chilled, you can cool the smoothie with a few ice cubes.

67. KALE PINEAPPLE SMOOTHIE

Prep Time: 3 Mins

Cook Time: 1 Mins

Total Time: 4 Mins

Servings: 2

Ingredients

- 2 cups of lightly packed sliced kale leaves, stems removed
- 1 frozen medium banana cut into chunks
- ¾ cup of unsweetened vanilla almond milk
- ¼ cup of plain non-fat Greek yogurt
- ¼ cup of frozen pineapple pieces
- 2 tbsp of creamy peanut butter
- 1-3 tsp of honey to taste

Instructions

1. In a blender, combine all the ingredients (kale, almond milk, banana, yogurt, pineapple, peanut butter, and honey) in the order given.
2. Blend until completely smooth. As needed, add more milk to get the appropriate consistency. Enjoy right now.

Notes

1. This kale smoothie tastes best right away, but it may be chilled for up to 4 hours (best results) or up to 1 day (less optimal results).

68. BROCCOLI SMOOTHIE RECIPE (TROPICAL AND VEGAN)

Prep Time: 5 Mins

Cook Time: 1 Mins

Total Time: 6 Mins

Servings: 2

Ingredients

- 2 cups of fresh pineapple chunks
- ½ cup of fresh baby spinach
- 1 cup of light coconut milk
- 1 cup of broccoli (frozen or fresh)
- 2 tbsp chia seeds (or hemp/chia)

Instructions

2. If you're new to smoothies, start with ½ cup of broccoli.
3. In a mixer, combine all ingredients, beginning with the liquid.
4. Mix until smooth, then slowly drink.
5. As needed, add extra liquid. Frozen veggies may require additional coconut milk.

69. TROPICAL SMOOTHIE RECIPE

Prep Time: 5 Mins

Cook Time: 1 Mins

Total Time: 6 Mins

Servings: 2

Ingredients

- ¾ cup of pineapple juice
- ½ cup of canned coconut milk
- 1 cup of frozen pineapple
- 1 large sliced banana
- 1 cup of frozen mango
- Optional garnishes: Maraschino cherries, mint sprigs, lime slices, pineapple wedges

Instructions

1. In a blender, mix the banana, pineapple juice, coconut milk, mango, and pineapple until totally smooth.
2. Place the smoothie in two glasses and decorate as desired.

70. ZUCCHINI DETOX SMOOTHIE

Total Time: 10 Mins

Servings: 1

Ingredients

- ¾ cup of green tea, at room temperature
- ½ cup of finely chopped zucchini
- ½ cup of finely chopped parsley
- 1 cup of finely chopped pineapple
- Juice of ½ lemon

Instructions

1. In a mixer, mix all the ingredients until they are entirely smooth.
2. Serve right away.

71. BERRY DETOX SMOOTHIE

Total Time: 10 Mins

Servings: 1

Ingredients

- 2 leaves of kale, rinsed, ribs removed and torn
- ⅓ cup of fresh blackberries
- ⅓ cup of fresh blueberries
- ⅓ cup of fresh raspberries
- 1 tbsp chia seeds
- 1 tbsp chopped walnuts
- 1 tbsp freshly squeezed lemon juice

- 1 tsp grated fresh ginger
- 1 cup of frozen strawberries
- ¾ cup of tart cherry juice
- Fresh fruit for garnish (optional)

Instructions

1. Combine all the ingredients in a mixer, except the fresh fruit, for garnish, and blend until smooth.
2. Put the smoothie into a glass and top with fresh fruit (if desired). Serve right away.

72. CHERRY BANANA SMOOTHIE

Total Time: 5 Mins

Servings: 1

Ingredients

- 1 cup of frozen cherries
- ½ banana
- 1 cup of almond milk
- ¼ cup of walnuts
- 1 tbsp hemp seeds
- 1 tsp Ceylon cinnamon
- Dash of ground cloves optional
- Toppings cacao nibs or chopped dark chocolate

Instructions

1. In a mixer, mix all the ingredients. Note: To make it easier to mix, add the wet ingredients first.
2. Mix everything on high speed until it's smooth and velvety.
3. A splash of milk or water may be added if the smoothie is too thick. Blend once more until everything is well mixed.
4. Like the smoothie and add more sugar if it's not sweet enough for your taste.
5. Get a smoothie glass and put the smoothie in it.
6. Add toppings: I used nibs of cacao. Be creative and add any toppings you choose.
7. Serving and having fun!

73. ANTI-INFLAMMATORY SMOOTHIE

Prep Time: 5 Mins

Cook Time: 45 Mins

Total Time: 50 Mins

Servings: 1

Ingredients

- ⅔ cup of beet, roasted, chopped, and frozen
- 2 cups of ripe strawberries, chopped and frozen
- 1 tsp fresh ginger, peeled and grated
- 1 tsp of fresh turmeric, peeled and grated
- 1 cup of unsweetened almond milk
- ½ cup of orange juice

Instructions

1. Begin by roasting or steaming your beet. I cut my beets into ½" pieces, wrapped them in foil, and cooked them for 40-45 minutes at 400 degrees. You may alternatively cut the beet in half and steam it for 15 to 20 minutes, or until it's tender when pricked with a fork.
2. After cooking your beet, let it cool, then put it in the freezer for at least two hours. Because you only need ⅔ cups, you could have extra roasted beet that you can use in salads.
3. Use a blender to mix all ingredients, then process them until they are completely smooth.
4. Serve with goji berries and full-fat coconut milk.

74. FRUIT CURRY

Total Time: 1 Hr 30 Mins

Servings: 6

Ingredients

- 2 onions
- ½ fresh pineapple
- ½ fresh small papaw
- 1 tbsp ghee or oil
- 1–2 tbsp of curry powder
- 1 peeled green apple
- 2 sliced bananas
- ¼ cup of desiccated coconut
- ⅔ cup of coconut milk
- ½ cup of sultanas
- 2 tbsp of soft brown sugar
- ½ tsp salt

Instructions

1. Slice the onion into 2.5 cm cubes. Chop the pineapple and papaw into 2.5 cm pieces.
2. In a big pan, heat the oil or ghee. Cook the onion until it is tender. Stir in the curry powder for 30 seconds, or until aromatic. Cook for 5 minutes, stirring gently, with the apple and pineapple.
3. Cook the papaw, bananas, coconut, and sultanas for 5 to 10 minutes, or until the fruit is cooked and the sauce has thickened somewhat.
4. Stir in the sugar and salt. Serve with steamed rice.

75. ORANGE SMOOTHIE

Total Time: 5 Mins

Servings: 1

Ingredients

- 2 large peeled oranges
- ½ tbsp orange zest
- 1 banana (room temperature)
- ¼ cup of Greek yogurt
- ½ tsp vanilla extract
- 1 tbsp of maple syrup (optional).
- 2 to 2 ½ cups of ice

Instructions

1. About ½ orange zest In a blender, combine the peeled oranges, orange zest, vanilla, Greek yogurt, banana, maple syrup or honey, and ice. Mix until completely smooth.
2. Enjoy immediately or chill for up to 1 day.

76. GRAPEFRUIT SMOOTHIE

Total Time: 10 Mins

Servings: 2

Ingredients

- 1 Winter Sweetz red grapefruit
- 2 cups of frozen pineapple chunks
- ⅓ cup of Greek yogurt
- 1 tbsp coconut oil
- ¼ inch knob of fresh ginger
- grapefruit segments, berries, and granola (for topping)

Instructions

1. Segment grapefruit over a bowl to catch all the juice. Set aside 2-3 segments for topping.

2. **Blend:** In a high-powered blender, combine grapefruit segments, grapefruit juice, frozen pineapple, Greek yogurt, coconut oil, and fresh ginger until smooth.
3. A splash of non-dairy milk may be added if the smoothie is excessively thick.
4. Pour into two glasses and serve. You may serve this in a bowl and top it with any toppings you like most, such as grapefruit segments, granola, berries, and so on.

77. BEETROOT AND CARROT SMOOTHIE

Total Time: 10 Mins

Servings: 2

Ingredients

- 1 cup of water
- 1 whole chopped beetroot
- 1 sliced carrot
- 1 cup of spinach
- 1 chopped small apple or pear
- 1 thin slice of ginger

Instructions

1. Chop and slice all of the fruits and vegetables roughly.
2. First, combine the water and spinach until smooth.
3. Then add the other ingredients and mix one more.
4. Pour into glasses to serve.

78. MANGO & KALE SMOOTHIE

Total time: 10 Mins

Servings: 1

Ingredients

- 1 cup of baby kale
- 1 cup of frozen mango chunks
- 1 small sliced banana
- 1 cup of fresh orange juice

Instructions

1. In a blender, combine the kale, mango, banana, and orange juice. Mix on medium-low speed, scraping down the sides as needed, until well combined.
2. Blend at a medium-high speed until the mixture is very smooth.

79. PEANUT BUTTER BANANA SMOOTHIE

Total Time: 5 Mins

Servings: 1

Ingredients

- 1 large banana sliced into chunks and frozen
- ¾ cup of unsweetened almond milk
- 2 tbsp of creamy peanut butter
- ½ cup of nonfat plain Greek yogurt
- ¼ tsp ground cinnamon
- Ice optional
- Optional mix-ins: ½ scoop protein powder (vanilla or chocolate) 1 tbsp flaxseed meal, 1 tbsp chia seeds

Instructions

1. In a blender, mix all ingredients in the order listed: almond milk, banana, peanut butter, Greek yogurt, cinnamon, and any extras.

2. Until smooth, blend, add a few ice cubes, and mix the smoothie once more if you want it thicker. Pour in and relish!

Notes

1. If you don't have a strong blender, you may need to add extra almond milk to achieve a smooth consistency. The frozen banana may be slowly added, blending in between each addition.
2. To keep For up to a day, store leftover smoothies in the refrigerator in airtight jars or containers.
3. To refrigerate For up to 3 months, you may freeze smoothies in freezer-safe jars or ice cube trays. Before serving, let the jars defrost in the fridge for a whole night. If using an ice cube tray on demand, place the frozen cubes into the blender for a smoothie on demand.

80. KIWI SMOOTHIES

Total Time: 10 Mins

Servings: 4

Ingredients

- 3 kiwifruit, peeled and cut into chunks
- 1 cup of fat-free plain yogurt
- 2 medium ripe bananas, slice into 4 pieces, and frozen
- 1 cup of frozen blueberries
- 3 tbsp of honey
- ¼ tsp almond extract, optional
- 1½ cups of crushed ice

Instructions

1. In a blender, add the fruit, yogurt, honey, and extract, if using, and blend until smooth. Add ice and process until smooth. If required, stir. Pour into cold glasses and serve right away.

81. WATERMELON SMOOTHIE

Total Time: 10 Mins

Servings: 1

Ingredients

- 150g of watermelon, peeled and chopped
- 1 small banana, peeled and sliced
- 100ml of cold apple juice

Instructions

2. Blend the watermelon, banana, and apple juice in a blender until smooth.
3. Serve the smoothie immediately in a large glass.

82. BEST GLOWING GREEN SMOOTHIE

Prep Time: 5 Mins

Servings: 2

Ingredients

- 1 large green apple
- 1 tbsp maple syrup
- ½ cup of water
- ¼ cup of raw cashews
- 3 cups of spinach
- 10 ice cubes
- 1 tbsp freshly squeezed lemon juice

Instructions

1. Leave the apple's peel on while you core and cut it into pieces.
2. Combine all the ingredients in a blender. Add the lemon juice and mix again for a few seconds. Taste and adjust with additional maple syrup or lemon juice as required. Serve immediately. Or refrigerate for up to 1 day.

83. BEST PEANUT BUTTER SMOOTHIE

Total Time: 5 Mins

Servings: 2

Ingredients

- 3 tbsp of peanut butter
- 2 medium ripe bananas (room temperature)
- ¾ cup of milk or non-dairy milk (like almond, oat, or coconut milk)
- 1 ½ cups of ice

Instructions

1. Mix all ingredients in a mixer, breaking the banana into pieces. Mix until completely smooth.

Notes

1. Add ½ tsp vanilla essence if you like a stronger milkshake flavor (optional).

84. FROZEN FRUIT SMOOTHIES

Total Time: 5 Mins

Servings: 2

Ingredients

- 1 frozen banana, peeled and sliced
- 2 cups of frozen strawberries, raspberries, or cherries
- 1 cup of milk
- ½ cup of plain or vanilla yogurt
- ½ cup of freshly squeezed orange juice
- 2 to 3 tbsp of honey or to taste

Instructions

2. Blend all of the ingredients in a blender until smooth. Pour into serving glasses and serve.

3. Substitute 1 cup of rice milk for the milk and yogurt in non-dairy smoothies. Instead, instead of dairy, use soy yogurt or milk.

85. PERFECT BANANA SMOOTHIE

Prep Time: 5 Mins

Servings: 2

Ingredients

4. 2 medium ripe bananas (room temperature)
5. 1 ½ cups of ice
6. ¼ cup of Greek yogurt
7. ½ to ¾ cup of milk or nondairy milk (like almond, oat, or coconut milk)
8. Optional mix-ins: 1 tbsp peanut butter, ¼ tsp vanilla extract, 1 to 2 tbsp coconut or toasted coconut

Instructions

9. In a mixer, mix all ingredients, breaking the banana into pieces (start with ½ cup of milk, then add as needed). Stop and scraping down the sides as needed. Mix until creamy and foamy. Decorate with banana slices and toasted coconut if preferred. Serve right away, or keep it in a sealed jar in the refrigerator for up to 2 days.

Notes

10. Make it vegan: Use another ½ banana or vegan yogurt.

86. SIMPLE SMOOTHIE FORMULA

Total Time: 14 Mins

Servings: 1

Ingredients

- ½ –1 cup of strawberries
- 1 frozen banana
- ½ cup of yogurt
- ½ cup of liquid of choice
- 2–3 tbsp peanut butter (other nut or seed butter will also work here!)

Instructions

1. In a mixer, mix all the ingredients until smooth and creamy.
2. If necessary, add more liquid to start the blender running.
3. ENJOY!

Notes

1. Most other types of fruit will also work!
2. If you want a lighter smoothie, replace the banana with cauliflower.

87. PERFECT BERRY SMOOTHIE

Total Time: 5 Mins

Servings: 2 Small Smoothies

Ingredients

- 1 banana (room temperature)
- ½ cup of Greek yogurt
- 1 ½ tbsp each maple syrup and honey
- 2 cups of frozen mixed berries
- 1 ¼ cups of milk
- ½ cup of ice
- Optional add-ins: 1 tbsp of almond butter, ¼ tsp vanilla, fresh mint leaves or basil leaves

Instructions

1. Mix all the ingredients in a blender, breaking the banana into bits. Stopping and scraping down the sides as needed, mix until creamy and foamy. Garnish with a frozen strawberry and a mint leaf, if preferred. Serve immediately. Cover and refrigerate for 2 days.

Notes

1. Use vegan yogurt or another ½ banana if you are vegan.

88. MINTY PINEAPPLE SMOOTHIE

Prep Time: 10 Mins

Servings: 2

Ingredients

- 200g pineapple, cored, peeled, and cut into chunks
- 50g of baby spinach leaves
- a few mint leaves
- 25g oats
- 2 tbsp linseed
- handful of unsalted, unroasted cashew nuts
- fresh lime juice, to taste

Instructions

1. Mix all ingredients in a mixer with 200ml of water until smooth. If it's too thick, add more water (up to 400ml) until you get the right texture.

89. THE PERFECT SMOOTHIE FORMULA

Total Time: 5 Mins

Servings: 1 Smoothie

Ingredients

Base Formula

- 1 frozen banana
- 1 cup of frozen fruit (peaches, berries, pineapple, mango, etc.)
- 1 cup of fresh baby greens, loosely packed (spinach, kale, etc.)
- 1 cup of plain, unsweetened dairy or non-dairy milk

Optional Add-Ins

- ½ cup of Greek yogurt (adds probiotics, creaminess, and healthy fats)
- 2 tbsp of nuts, nut butter, or seeds (adds healthy fats)
- Sweetener, to taste (honey, maple syrup, stevia)
- 1-2 tbsp of nutrition boosts (protein powder, green powder, etc.)

Instructions

2. Put all of the ingredients in the mixer carafe in the order stated.
3. Blend all ingredients until smooth.

Notes

4. Don't like bananas? For a similar creamy result, use frozen avocado and a bit more sweetener. You can also get similar results from canned pears in juice and Greek yogurt. For additional ideas, see our list of no-banana smoothies!

90. STRAWBERRY BANANA SMOOTHIE

Total Time: 5 Mins

Servings: 3

Ingredients

- 1 ½ cups of raspberries
- 1 cup of strawberries
- ½ frozen banana
- 1 cup of almond milk, or oat milk
- 1 tbsp honey or maple syrup
- 1 ½ cups of ice
- Handful of mint or basil, optional

Instructions

1. In a blender, mix the raspberries, strawberries, banana, almond milk, honey or maple, basil, if using, and ice. Blend until completely smooth.
2. Taste. If it's too sour, add another ½ cup of almond milk and another tbsp honey or maple syrup.

Notes

1. Optional step, strain to remove seeds: Mix all ingredients except for the ice. Drain the liquid to remove the strawberry seeds, then return it to the blender with the ice and pulse until mixed.

91. BANANA, CLEMENTINE & MANGO SMOOTHIE

Prep Time: 15-25 Mins

Servings: 6

Ingredients

- 24 juicy clementines plus one extra for decorating
- 500g tub whole milk or low-fat yogurt
- 2 small, very ripe, and juicy mangoes
- 2 ripe bananas
- handful of ice cubes (optional)

Instructions

1. Cut the clementines in half and squeeze off the juice; you should have around 600ml (1 pint). (You may do this the night before.) Peel the mangoes, then cut the fruit away from the center stone and chop the flesh into rough pieces. Bananas, peeled and sliced

2. In a liquidizer, mix the clementine juice, mango flesh, bananas, yogurt, and ice cubes and blend until smooth. Pour the mixture into six glasses and serve. (Depending on the size of your liquidizer, you may need to prepare this in two batches.) If no ice cubes are used, chill in the refrigerator until ready to serve.

92. PERFECT PEACH SMOOTHIE

Total Time: 5 Mins

Servings: 2

Ingredients

- 2 cups of peaches, frozen (or fresh, and use a frozen banana)
- ¼ cup of Greek yogurt
- 1 banana (room temperature)
- ½ tbsp maple syrup, honey, or agave syrup
- 1 cup of milk
- 6 ice cubes
- ½ tsp vanilla extract
- ¼ tsp cinnamon

Instructions

1. In a mixer, mix all the ingredients, breaking the banana into pieces. Stopping and scraping down the sides as needed, blend until creamy and foamy. Garnish with a frozen peach if desired. Serve immediately, cover, and refrigerate for 1 day.

Notes

1. Vegan yogurt can be substituted. Prepare a Peach Banana Smoothie: 2 cups of frozen peaches, 2 bananas (room temperature), ½ cup of water, and 8 ice cubes with the same quantity of vanilla and cinnamon.

93. MOZZARELLA SOUP WITH VEGETABLES AND OLIVES

Total Time: 45 Mins

Servings: 4

Ingredients

- 3 tbsp of extra virgin olive oil
- 2 small celery ribs, very coarsely sliced
- 1 large peeled and roughly sliced red onion
- 8 ounces of peeled baby-cut fresh carrots, very coarsely chopped
- 1 large baking potato, peeled and diced
- 1 large minced garlic clove
- 1 whole bay leaf
- 1 sprig of fresh rosemary (3 inches) or ½ tsp dried rosemary, crumbled
- 14 ½ ounces of canned chicken broth
- 12 ounces of canned evaporated milk (use skim if you like)
- ½ cup of fresh whole milk
- ½ tsp hot red pepper sauce
- 4 ounces of finely shredded mozzarella cheese
- ⅓ cup of sliced pitted ripe olives
- salt & freshly ground black pepper

Instructions

2. 1 minute over medium heat, heat oil in a large, heavy saucepan.
3. Cook, often stirring, for 5 minutes, with the onion, carrots, celery, potato, garlic, bay leaf, and rosemary.
4. Reduce heat to low, cover, and allow veggies to "sweat" for 10 minutes.
5. Bring broth to a gentle boil, then cover and cook until potato is cooked about 15 minutes.
6. Remove the bay leaf and rosemary sprig; bring the evaporated milk, milk, and red pepper sauce to a boil.
7. Remove from heat and mix in mozzarella until smooth.
8. Stir in the olives and season with salt and pepper to taste.
9. Pour into heated soup bowls and serve.

94. PASTA WITH CAPERS, OLIVES AND PINE NUTS

Prep time: 10 Mins

Cook time: 15 Mins

Total time: 25 Mins

Servings: 6

Ingredients

- 3 tbsp of butter
- 3 ounces of olive oil
- 3 minced garlic cloves
- 3 ounces of pine nuts
- 15 ounces of sliced California black olives
- 3 tbsp of capers (rinsed and minced)
- 1 tbsp basil (cut into chiffonade)
- 1 tsp minced oregano
- 1 tsp minced flat parsley
- 1 pound of pasta (any shape)
- Salt (to taste)
- Ground black pepper (to taste)
- 2 ounces of grated Parmesan cheese

Instructions

1. Get the ingredients.
2. In a large saute pan, mix the butter and olive oil and heat over medium heat.
3. Become down the heat to low and simmer the pine nuts until they begin to turn a golden brown color.
4. Combine the olives, capers, basil, oregano, parsley, salt, and pepper in a mixing bowl. Mix until all ingredients are incorporated and completely hot.
5. Cook the pasta until al dente in a big pot of boiling salted water. Drain thoroughly. Over medium heat, toss the cooked, drained pasta with the nut-olive mixture until well combined and heated. To taste, season with salt and black pepper.
6. Add grated Parmesan cheese to each serving.

95. HEALTHY MOUSSAKA

Prep Time: 45 Mins

Cook Time: 45 Mins

Total Time: 1 Hr 30 Mins

Servings: 12 Slices

Ingredients

For the meat sauce

- Olive oil cooking spray
- 1 large white or red onion
- 3 garlic cloves, minced
- 750g of extra lean beef mince
- 2 tbsp sweetener (Sukrin Gold)
- 2 tsp cinnamon
- 1 tsp salt
- Pinch ground cloves
- 1 tsp dried thyme
- 1 bay leaf
- 2 tbsp Worcestershire sauce
- 1 tbsp soy sauce or tamari
- 1 tsp fish sauce (optional)
- 100g tomato paste (purée)
- 400g Passata
- 300ml hot beef stock made with 2 stock cubes

For the aubergine layer

- Olive oil cooking spray
- 3 large aubergines (eggplants)
- Salt

For the topping

- 1 tbsp low fat spread
- 2 tbsp flour
- 450g fat-free Greek yogurt

- 200g Greek feta, crumbled (sub with fat-free cottage cheese)
- 3 eggs, lightly beaten
- Salt and pepper
- Pinch of freshly ground nutmeg
- 2 tbsp grated Parmesan (optional)

Instructions

1. Prepare the meat sauce.
2. Spray a skillet or casserole lightly with olive oil or low-calorie cooking spray. Cook, occasionally stirring, for five minutes over low heat with the onions and garlic.
3. Break up the minced beef with the back of a wooden spoon. Brown the meat for a few minutes or until it is nicely browned.
4. Mix the salt, sugar (I used Sukrin Gold), thyme, cinnamon, cloves, and bay leaf in a mixing bowl.
5. Mix the tomato puree (paste), passata, soy, fish, and Worcestershire sauces in a mixing bowl.
6. Bring to a simmer with the beef stock. Cook over medium heat for 30 minutes, stirring every now and then, or until the sauce thickens and the liquid reduces.
7. Remove the bay leaf. Sprinkle the sauce with salt and pepper as required.
8. Make the aubergine (eggplant)
9. While the beef sauce is simmering, cut the aubergine either widthwise or in rounds. The slices must be around 1 centimeter thick or a bit thinner. Sprinkle with salt, olive oil, or a low-calorie cooking spray like Fry light.
10. Cook the aubergine on a griddle pan for 3-4 minutes per side. Alternatively, preheat the broiler (grill) to high. Cook the pieces for 8–10 minutes on each side, or until tender. Don't let them burn! While you make the topping, place the aubergine on paper towels.

Notes

1. Tips for Making the Best Moussaka Ever!
2. You may make the meat sauce up to a day ahead of time. You don't want a runny sauce ruining your moussaka, so make sure the sauce is thick.
3. Season the cheese sauce to taste. Even though feta cheese adds a lot of flavors, you should still season the sauce with salt, pepper, and freshly grated nutmeg.
4. Before layering the aubergine slices (or any other vegetable) into the casserole, make sure they are soft.

5. Instead of or in addition to aubergines, you may cook potatoes or squash in a single layer on a baking tray for 30 minutes at 350F or until they are tender when poked with a fork. Sprinkle with salt and spray with olive oil.
6. Rest the cooked moussaka for at least 15-20 minutes before slicing. It need this time to cool slightly and firm up enough to cut.
7. Moussaka stays in the fridge for 3-4 days and tastes even better the next day! Before serving, reheat in the microwave until well warmed.

96. MOUSSAKA: EGGPLANT CASSEROLE

Prep Time: 20 Mins

Cook Time: 1 Hr 30 Mins

Total Time: 1 Hr 50 Mins

Servings: 12 Pieces

Ingredients

- 2 large eggplants, sliced lengthwise into ¼-inch-thick slices, end slices discarded
- salt
- Private Reserve extra virgin olive oil
- 4 tbsp of breadcrumbs

For the meat sauce

- 1 large finely chopped yellow onion
- 1 pound of ground lamb or beef
- 1 tbsp dried oregano
- 1 tsp ground cinnamon
- ½ tsp black pepper
- ½ tsp ground nutmeg
- ½ tsp paprika or hot paprika
- ½ cup of red wine
- 14-ounce can of diced tomato
- 1 tsp sugar
- ½ cup of hot beef broth

For the bechamel

- ⅓ cup + 2 tbsp extra virgin olive oil
- ⅔ cup of all-purpose flour
- ½ tsp salt, more if you like
- ¼ tsp ground nutmeg
- 4 cups of warmed milk
- 2 large eggs

Instructions

1. Salt the eggplant. Spread the eggplant slices out in a single layer and season with salt. Allow to stand for 30 minutes to "sweat off" the bitterness.
2. Turn on your oven's broiler.
3. Brush a large sheet pan or two with extra virgin olive oil. Remove any excess salt from the eggplant slices and lay them in a single layer on the prepared pan. Brush with olive oil liberally.
4. Set the sheet pan 6 inches away from the broiler. Cook the eggplant for a few minutes, turning it over until both sides are soft and brown (don't worry if some of the eggplant is slightly charred, but keep an eye on it, so it doesn't burn). Remove from the oven and put aside.
5. Make the meat sauce. 2 tbsp of olive oil, heated in a pan. Cook the onions over medium heat, often stirring, until they turn slightly golden brown (about 5 minutes). Now mix in the ground lamb. Cook the lamb until it is completely browned, tossing often. Drain the lamb of any extra fat and put it back in the pan. Combine the dried oregano, cinnamon, pepper, nutmeg, and hot paprika in a bowl. Stir in the spices to coat the meat. Boil for 1 minute to reduce the wine. Combine the canned tomatoes, sugar, and broth in a bowl. Cook for 20 to 30 minutes on medium-low heat.
6. Meanwhile, preheat the oven to 350°F and resume work on the bechamel.
7. Make the bechamel. In a large saucepan, place the olive oil and heat it over medium-high heat until it shimmers but does not start to smoke. Mix the salt, flour, and pepper in a bowl. Cook until golden brown (if needed, add a little more olive oil). Whisk continuously as you gradually add the hot milk. Cook for five to seven minutes, stirring the mixture regularly, over medium heat. Mix in the nutmeg. In a bowl, mix 2 eggs and a small amount of the heated bechamel mixture. Then return everything to the pan and mix it into the bechamel sauce. Continue to stir or whisk the mixture while bringing it to a gentle boil for 2 minutes. Adjust the seasoning to taste. Let it chill and thicken a bit more after removing from the heat. (A creamy, thick, and smooth bechamel sauce should result.)
8. Make the moussaka. When ready, lightly spray a 9 ½" x 13" oven-safe baking dish with cooking spray. Put half of the eggplant slices on the bottom. Spread the meat

sauce evenly. Finish with the remaining eggplant pieces. Spread the bechamel equally over the eggplant, then sprinkle with the bread crumbs.

9. Bake. Bake the moussaka casserole for 45 minutes on the middle rack of a preheated oven. Transfer the baking pan to the top rack and broil briefly to get a wonderful golden brown color on the top of the moussaka (watch carefully).

10. Take it off the heat and let it aside for 10 minutes before cutting it into squares to serve. Enjoy!

Notes

1. You may make and broil the eggplant and meat sauce a day or two ahead of time. The bechamel sauce can also be made ahead of time (it can hold texture for about 1 week, although you should count some days for leftovers). If you prepare the eggplant casserole components ahead of time, store them in separate, tightly closed containers in the refrigerator. If the bechamel thickens too much, reheat it gently over low heat before using, adding a little additional milk and stirring to ensure the mixture is not lumpy.

2. Allow the moussaka to rest for 10 to 20 minutes before serving: After taking the eggplant moussaka from the oven, set it aside for 10 to 20 minutes to allow the bechamel sauce to settle.

3. Moussaka will keep in the fridge for about five days (although you need to count any make-ahead days).

4. Cooked moussaka may be frozen. Once the moussaka is entirely cool, just cut it into pieces and put them in separate containers that can go in the freezer, or wrap each piece tightly in parchment paper and then foil. You may reheat individual slices at a time this way.

97. CREAMY CARROT AND TURNIP SOUP

Prep Time: 10 Mins

Cook Time: 30 Mins

Total Time: 40 Mins

Servings: 4

Ingredients

- 4 large carrots
- 1 potato
- 1 tbsp butter
- 1 tbsp olive oil
- 1 leek
- 2 minced garlic cloves
- 3 medium chopped turnips
- salt and black pepper, to taste
- 2 cups of vegetable broth or water
- 1 cup of heavy cream
- chopped parsley, for garnish

Instructions

1. Bring water in a pot to a full boil. Cook the carrots and potatoes for 20 to 25 minutes, or until the carrots are soft.
2. Meanwhile, cut the leek into slices, removing the dark green leaf end and the root end (only utilize the white and light green sections). Add the leek to a hot pan with butter and olive oil. Cook for around 4-5 minutes.
3. Cook for 30 seconds additional, or until the garlic is aromatic. Cook for 5 minutes more after adding the turnips. Cook for a few minutes more after adding the cooked carrots and potatoes. Sprinkle with salt and pepper.
4. Mix the veggies with the broth in a blender. Mix until well combined. Pour the mixture into the pot you used to cook the carrots. Mix in the heavy cream and add salt and pepper to taste. Bring it to a boil, then remove it from the heat.
5. Garnish with chopped parsley before serving.

98. CROCK POT BEEF AND CHICKEN STEW

Prep Time: 20 Mins

Cook Time: 8 Hrs

Total Time: 8 Hrs 20 Mins

Servings: 8

Ingredients

- 3 tbsp steak sauce
- 2 chicken bouillon cubes
- 1 tsp kosher salt
- ½ tsp freshly ground black pepper
- 1 tsp sugar
- ½ cup of hot water or stock
- 2 pounds of boneless, skinless chicken thighs
- 1 pound lean stewing beef, cut into ½ -inch cubes
- ½ cup of chopped onion
- 2 medium peeled and cubed potatoes
- 2 medium carrots, peeled and thinly sliced
- 14 ½ ounce fo stewed tomatoes
- ¼ cup of all-purpose flour

Instructions

1. Get the ingredients.
2. In a slow cooker, mix the steak sauce, bouillon cubes, salt, pepper, sugar, and boiling water. To combine the ingredients, stir them together.
3. Mix the chicken thighs, meat, onion, potatoes, carrots, and tomatoes in a large bowl. Gently stir.
4. Cook for 8-10 hours on low or 5 hours on high.
5. Take the chicken thighs halfway through the cooking time. Cut them up and put the meat back in the slow cooker. Finish cooking by stirring well.
6. Prepare a smooth paste with the flour and ¼ cup of cold water to thicken the gravy. In the slow cooker, mix in the flour mixture. Simmer for about 15-20 minutes on high, or until thickened.
7. Serve with crusty toast, biscuits, or cornbread.
8. Enjoy.

99. PUMPKIN SOUP - CLASSIC AND EASY

Prep Time: 5 Mins

Cook Time: 10 Mins

Total Time: 15 Mins

Servings: 8

Ingredients

- 2.4-pound pumpkin, unpeeled weight (Note 1)
- 1 sliced onion (white, brown, yellow)
- 2 garlic cloves, peeled whole
- 750ml vegetable or chicken broth or stock, low sodium
- 250ml water
- Salt and pepper

Finishes

- 125–185 ml of cream, half and half, or milk

Instructions

1. Cut the pumpkin into 3cm (2.25") slices. Remove the skin and scrape out the seeds (video is helpful). 4cm/1.5" slices into "chunks.
2. In a pot, mix the pumpkin, onion, garlic, broth, and water; the liquid will not completely cover the pumpkin. Bring to a boil, uncovered, then decrease heat and let simmer for 10 minutes, or until pumpkin is soft (check with a butter knife).
3. Take off the heat and mix with a stick blender until smooth (Note 3 for blender).
4. Sprinkle with salt to taste, then fold in the cream (never boil the soup after adding soup, cream will split).
5. Drizzle soup into bowls, top with cream, and top with pepper and parsley, if preferred. Serve with crusty bread!

Notes

1. Pumpkin - 2.4-pound pumpkin before peeling and seeds.
2. You'll need two cans of canned pumpkin puree to prepare this. Cream - Adding a layer of richness to the mouthfeel using cream. But it's still great even without - I frequently make it with only milk. Instead, I sometimes stir in a touch of butter for a richer finish!

3. Pureeing-you can use a blender, but make sure the soup is slightly cooled before mixing it, otherwise, you will learn the hard way that hot soup + blender = soup explosion (literally, the lid will blow off the blender when you start blending it).

100. BUTTERY ONION SOUP

Prep Time: 5 Mins

Cook Time: 30 Mins

Total Time: 35 Mins

Servings: 6

Ingredients

- 2 cups of thinly sliced onions
- ½ cup of cubed butter
- ¼ cup of all-purpose flour
- 2 cups of chicken broth
- 2 cups of milk
- 1- ½ to 2 cups of shredded part-skim mozzarella cheese
- Salt and pepper to taste
- Croutons, optional

Instructions

1. Cook onions in butter in a large pan over low heat until soft and translucent, around 20 minutes.
2. Mix in the flour. Cook and mix the broth and milk over medium heat until bubbly. Cook and stir for another 1 minute, then reduce to low heat. Mix in the mozzarella cheese until it is completely melted (do not boil). Sprinkle with salt to taste. If necessary, serve with croutons.

101. ASPARAGUS SOUP

Prep Time: 10 Mins

Cook Time: 20 Mins

Total Time: 30 Mins

Servings: 4

Ingredients

- 25g of butter
- a little vegetable oil
- 3 finely sliced shallots
- 350g stalks chopped, asparagus spear, woody ends discarded, tips reserved
- 2 crushed garlic cloves
- 2 large handfuls of spinach
- 700ml vegetable stock (fresh if possible)
- olive oil, for drizzling (optional)
- rustic bread (preferably sourdough), to serve (optional)

Instructions

1. Warm the butter and oil in a Big saucepan until foamy. Soften the asparagus tips in a pan for a few minutes. Take it out and set it aside.
2. Simmer for 5–10 minutes until the shallots, asparagus stalks, and garlic are softened but still bright. Mix in the spinach, then pour in the stock, bring to a boil, and blitz with a hand mixer.
3. Season thoroughly and, if necessary, add hot water to loosen. Pour into serving bowls and top with asparagus tips. If desired, drizzle with olive oil and serve over sourdough bread.

102. CHEESEBURGER SOUP

Prep Time: 15 Mins

Cook Time: 30 Mins

Total Time: 45 Mins

Servings: 6

Ingredients

- 1 pound ground beef
- ¾ cup of chopped onion
- ¾ cup of shredded carrots
- ¾ cup of diced celery
- 1 tsp dried basil
- 1 tsp dried parsley flakes
- 4 tbsp butter divided
- 3 cups of chicken broth
- 4 cups of peeled and diced potatoes
- ¼ cup of all purpose flour
- 2 cups of cheese cubed
- 1 ½ cups of milk
- ¾ tsp salt
- ¼ to ½ tsp pepper
- ¼ cup of sour cream

Instructions

1. In a 3 quart pot, brown the ground beef. Drain and set aside.
2. 1 tbsp butter, onion, shredded carrots, parsley flakes, basil, and celery in the same pan Cook until tender.
3. Bring the broth, potatoes, and beef to a boil. Reduce the heat to low, cover, and cook for 10-12 minutes, or until the potatoes are soft.
4. Melt the remaining butter (3 T) in a small pan and stir in the flour. Cook the mixture while stirring it for three to five minutes, or until it begins to bubble. Bring to a boil with the soup. Cook for 2 minutes, stirring frequently. Reduce the heat to low.
5. Add the cheese, milk, salt, and pepper to taste. Cook, stirring constantly, until the cheese melts. Trun off the heat and stir in the sour cream.

103. COD FISH SOUP

Prep Time: 10 Mins

Cook Time: 25 Mins

Total Time: 35 Mins

Servings: 6

Ingredients

- 12 ounces cod fillets
- 9 cups of water
- 3 medium chopped potatoes
- 2 thinly sliced carrots
- ½ medium finely chopped onion
- 2 thinly sliced celery stalks
- 2 tbsp of avocado oil
- 1 minced garlic clove
- 1 bay leaf
- 2 tbsp parsley (fresh)
- 1 tbsp lemon juice
- salt
- pepper

Instructions

1. Bring to boil the water in a saucepan.
2. Chop the potatoes. Cut celery and carrots into thin slices. Chop the onion finely.
3. Bring the potatoes and carrots back to a boil in the water. Lid and cook for 10 minutes on low heat.
4. Heat the avocado oil in a pan. Cook for 7 minutes with celery and onion. Pour into the pot.
5. Chop the fish and mince the garlic; add them to the soup.
6. Combine the parsley, bay leaf, and lemon juice in a bowl. Sprinkle with salt and pepper. Cook the fish for approximately 7 minutes or until it is fully cooked.
7. With toasted bread, serve.

104. BEEF AND MACARONI SOUP

Prep Time: 15 Mins

Cook Time: 20 Mins

Total Time: 35 Mins

Servings: 6

Ingredients

- 1 pound lean ground beef
- ½ cup of diced onion
- 6 cups of beef broth
- 14 ounces diced tomatoes
- 2 tbsp tomato paste
- 1 tsp Worcestershire sauce
- ½ tsp oregano
- ½ tsp dried basil
- 1 ½ cups of elbow macaroni uncooked
- 1 ½ cups of frozen mixed vegetables

Instructions

1. In a big soup pot, brown the beef and onion until there is no pinker. Drain all fat.
2. Add the spices, broth, tomatoes, tomato paste, and Worcestershire sauce. Bring to a simmer. Simmer 5 minutes.
3. Add macaroni and veggies, and continue simmering for an additional 8 minutes, or until macaroni is cooked. Season to taste with salt and pepper.
4. If preferred, serve with shredded cheese.

Notes

1. If adding fresh veggies, add them before the pasta so they can soften.
2. If you will not eat all of this in one sitting, prepare the pasta separately and put it to separate bowls. If the macaroni is left overnight in the soup, it will soak the broth and become mushy.
3. Change the taste of this soup by adding seasonings and toppings. For a taco soup, try taco seasoning with avocados, sliced jalapenos, and a dollop of sour cream on top.
4. Substitute black beans for the ground beef, pinto beans, or black-eyed peas for a vegetarian option.

5. For optimal results when freezing pasta, leave it out and add it while reheating.

105. BEEF ENCHILADA SOUP

Prep Time: 10 Mins

Cook Time: 20 Mins

Total Time: 30 Mins

Servings: 8

Ingredients

- 2-pound lean ground beef
- 3 tbsp taco seasoning
- 1 onion
- 2 cans of red enchilada sauce
- 1 jar Zoup! Beef Bone Broth
- 1 can of diced tomatoes not drained
- 1 can of sweet corn drained
- 1 can of black beans not drained
- 1 can green chiles not drained
- Toppings (optional)
- Corn tortillas cut into strips
- Sour cream
- Cheddar cheese shredded
- diced Cilantro

Instructions

1. Combine the ground beef, taco seasoning, and chopped onion in a skillet. Simmer over medium-high heat until the meat is no longer pink. Discard any extra grease or liquid.
2. Enchilada sauce, tomatoes, corn, black beans, green chiles, Zoup Beef Bone Broth, and stir to blend. Cover and simmer for 10 minutes.
3. Serve hot with sour cream, cheddar cheese, chopped Cilantro, and pieces of corn tortilla.

106. SERIOUSLY GOOD VEGETABLE SOUP

Prep Time: 15 Mins

Cook Time: 45 Mins

Total Time: 1 Hr

Servings: 6 bowls

Ingredients

- 4 tbsp extra-virgin olive oil, divided
- 1 medium chopped yellow onion
- 3 peeled and chopped carrots
- 2 chopped celery stalks
- 2 cups of chopped seasonal vegetables
- 1 large can of diced tomatoes
- 1 tsp fine sea salt (to taste)
- ½ tsp curry powder
- 6 cloves garlic, pressed or minced
- ½ tsp dried thyme
- 4 cups of vegetable broth
- 2 bay leaves
- 2 cups of water
- Freshly ground black pepper, to taste
- ½ tsp red pepper flakes, reduced or omitted if spice sensitive
- 1 tbsp lemon juice
- 2 cups of sliced kale or collard greens or chard (thick ribs removed)

Instructions

1. In a large Dutch oven or soup pot, heat 3 tbsp olive oil over medium heat. Add the onion, carrot, celery, seasonal vegetables, and ½ tsp salt as the oil begins to shimmer. Cook, often stirring, for 6 to 8 minutes, or until the onion has softened and turned translucent.
2. Mix the garlic, curry powder, and thyme in a bowl. Cook until aromatic, approximately 1 minute, stirring frequently. Add the sliced tomatoes with their juices and keep cooking, often stirring, for a few more minutes.
3. Add the broth and water. Add ½ tsp additional salt, 2 bay leaves, and red pepper flakes to taste. To taste, season with freshly ground black pepper. Raise the heat to

bring the mixture to a boil, then reduce to a slow simmer by partially cover the saucepan.

4. After 25 minutes, remove the top and stir in the chopped greens. Continue to boil for 5 minutes or until the greens are soft enough to your liking.
5. Take the bay leaves from the saucepan and set aside. Combine the lemon juice and the remaining 1 tbsp of olive oil in a bowl. Sprinkle with more salt, pepper, or red pepper flakes to taste. (Depending on your veggie broth and personal preferences, you may need up to ½ tsp extra salt.) Serve in bowls and enjoy.

Notes

1. **Storage suggestions:** This soup will keep in the fridge for approximately 4 days. If you want to save additional pieces for later, it freezes and defrosts well!

107. CREAMY POTATO & HAMBURGER SOUP

Prep Time: 20 Mins

Cook Time: 4 Hrs

Total Time: 4 Hrs 20 Mins

Servings: 10

Ingredients

- 1 ½ pounds lean ground beef
- 1 medium peeled and diced white onion
- 1 large minced garlic clove
- 6 cups of chicken broth
- 2 cups of frozen vegetable mix of your choice
- 6 cups of peeled & diced Russet potatoes
- 3 tsp dried basil
- 2 tsp dried parsley flakes
- 1 ½ cups of milk
- 2 tbsp cornstarch
- 8 ounces Velveeta cheese cubed

Instructions

1. Fry the ground beef and onions in a large pan until the onions are tender and the ground beef is browned. Remove the grease.
2. Fry the garlic until it is golden and fragrant. Add the meat mixture to the crockpot or stockpot on the stove.
3. Combine the potatoes, broth, veggies, basil, and parsley in a bowl.
4. Cook on low for 6-8 hours, then increase the heat to high for 3-4 hours or simmer until the potatoes are tender and starting to melt slightly.
5. Stir the cornstarch into the milk before adding it to the soup. Allow the Velveeta to melt, stirring frequently. When it's all melted in, spoon it into bowls and serve.

Notes

2. Add broth thins soup or ½ cup of sour cream towards the end to give some tang.

108. BASIC HAM AND BEAN SOUP

Prep Time: 30 Mins

Cook Time: 2 Hrs 30 Mins

Total Time: 3 Hrs

Servings: 9

Ingredients

- 1 pound dry great Northern beans
- 8 cups of water
- ½ tsp salt
- 1 ham hock
- 1 cup of chopped carrots
- ½ chopped stalk celery
- 1 cup of chopped onion
- 1 tsp minced garlic
- 1 tsp mustard powder
- 2 bay leaves
- 2 cups of chopped ham
- ½ tsp ground white pepper

Instructions

3. Rinse the beans, removing any broken or discolored ones. Bring to boil the water in a big saucepan over high heat. Take from the fire after adding the salt and beans. Allow beans to soak in boiling water for at least 60 minutes.
4. After 60 minutes, return the pot to high heat and add the ham bone, carrots, celery, onion, garlic, mustard, and bay leaves. Mix thoroughly, bring to a boil, then lower to low heat and continue to cook for 60 minutes.
5. Discard the ham bone. Simmer for about 30 minutes after adding the chopped ham. To taste, sprinkle with ground white pepper.

109. BEEFY MEXICAN RICE SOUP

Prep Time: 15 Mins

Cook Time: 45 Mins

Total Time 1 Hr

Servings: 10

Ingredients

- 2 pounds of ground beef
- ⅓ cup of chopped onion
- 1 tsp minced garlic
- 3 tbsp taco seasoning
- 2 quarts of beef stock
- 2 cups of frozen corn
- 15.5 ounces black beans (rinsed and drained)
- 14.5 ounces petite diced tomatoes (drained)
- 1 cup of tomato puree
- 2 tsp lime juice
- 2 tsp salt
- 1 tsp cilantro
- 1 cup of whole grain rice

Instructions

1. Brown the ground beef, onion, and chopped garlic in a large dutch oven. Drain.
2. Combine the taco seasoning and stir well.

3. Combine the beef stock, corn, black beans, diced tomatoes, tomato puree, lime juice, salt, cilantro, and rice in a large bowl.
4. Bring to a boil, then lid and cook for 25-30 minutes, or until the rice is tender.
5. If preferred, top with cheese, sour cream, and cilantro.

110. CREAMY GREEK YOGURT PASTA

Prep Time: 10 Mins

Cook Time: 15 Mins

Total Time: 25 Mins

Servings: 6

Ingredients

- 3 large lemons
- 1 ¾ ounce
- Finely grated Parmesan cheese
- ½ bunch fresh parsley, optional
- 1 pound dried fettuccine pasta
- 1 ½ cups of full-fat plain Greek yogurt
- 3 cloves garlic
- 3 tbsp
- extra-virgin olive oil
- 1 tsp freshly ground black pepper
- ½ tsp kosher salt

Instructions

1. Over high heat, bring a big pot of heavily salted water to a boil. Meanwhile, combine the following ingredients in a blender: finely grate the zest and juice of 3 big lemons; finely grate 1 ¾ ounces Parmesan cheese (about 1 cup). Set aside the leaves from ½ bunch of fresh parsley for garnishing if using.
2. Cook until al dente, approximately 8 minutes, or according to package instructions, 1 pound of dry fettuccine in boiling water. Meanwhile, in a blender, combine 1 ½ cups of Greek yogurt, 3 tbsp extra-virgin olive oil, 1 tsp black pepper, 3 garlic cloves, and ½ tsp kosher salt. Blend on high for 2 minutes, or until the Parmesan cheese is completely absorbed and the sauce is smooth.
3. Remove and return the fettucine to the pot when it is done. Pour in the yogurt mixture and thoroughly toss and combine the sauce with tongs. The sauce will be

thin at first, but it will thicken as the cheese melts. Season with salt and pepper to taste. If preferred, sprinkle with chopped parsley and serve warm.

111. MACARONI SALAD WITH TOMATOES

Prep Time: 15 Mins

Cook Time: 10 Mins

Total Time: 25 Mins

Servings: 7

Ingredients

- 6 ounce uncooked elbows (wheat or gluten-free)
- 2 medium diced tomatoes
- ¼ finely chopped red onion
- ¼ cup of light mayonnaise
- 1 tbsp white vinegar
- dash garlic powder
- 1 tsp oregano
- 2.5 ounce sliced black olives
- salt and pepper

Instructions

1. Cook the pasta in salted water as direct on the box.
2. Drain and rinse with cool water.
3. Mix mayonnaise, vinegar, tomatoes (and any liquid from the tomatoes), olives, onion, garlic powder, oregano, salt, and pepper in a medium mixing bowl. Combine thoroughly.
4. Mix in the elbows well.

112. EGG SALAD WITH OLIVES RECIPE

Total Time: 10 Mins

Servings: 6

Ingredients

- 6 hard-cooked eggs
- ¼ cup of mayonnaise
- salt and ground black pepper to taste
- ¼ cup of sliced green olives stuffed with pimentos
- ¼ cup of diced sweet onion

Instructions

1. In a big bowl or your stand mixer's bowl, mash the eggs with a fork or the paddle attachment of your stand mixer. Add mayonnaise and stir until well-combined and eggs are light and airy. Add to taste salt and ground black pepper.
2. Stir olives, pimentos, and onion slices into the egg salad.

113. CHICKEN TACO SALAD

Total Time: 16 Mins

Servings: 6

Ingredients

- 2 boneless, skinless chicken breasts
- 2 tbsp taco seasoning
- ¼ cup of vegetable oil
- 2 tbsp butter

Dressing

- ¾ cup of ranch dressing
- ¼ cup of salsa
- 3 tbsp finely minced fresh cilantro

Salad

- 2 ears of corn, shucked
- 1 large head or 2 regular heads of green leaf lettuce, shredded thin
- 3 diced Roma tomatoes
- ½ cup of grated pepper-jack cheese
- 2 diced avocados
- 3 sliced green onions
- Crushed tortilla chips of your choosing (flavored or unflavored) for salad topper
- ½ cup of fresh cilantro leaves

Instructions

1. To prepare the chicken, generously season both sides of the breasts with taco seasoning. Warm the oil and butter in a big skillet over medium-high heat. Cook the chicken for 4 minutes on each side, or until deep golden brown on the outside and done in the center (or to an internal temperature of 165 degrees F). Set aside for 5 minutes to cool.
2. Pour the ranch dressing into a bowl and set aside while the chicken cooks. Stir in the salsa and cilantro to mix.
3. To make the salad, place the ears of corn in the pan you used to cook the chicken and roll them around to coat them with the flavorful oil/butter mixture. Grill the corn on a grill pan until it is crisp but has color on the outside. Using a sharp knife, remove the kernels and put them aside. Cut the chicken into cubes.
4. Layer the shredded lettuce, diced chicken, tomatoes, cheese, corn, avocados, green onions, cilantro, and smashed chips on a platter. Drizzle the dressing over the top, reserving some for serving on the side if desired. Serve the salad in individual bowls.

114. CLASSIC COLESLAW

Prep Time: 25 Mins

Cook Time: 1 Hr

Total Time: 1 Hr 25 Mins

Servings: 10

Ingredients

- 1 small head of green cabbage
- ½ small head of red cabbage
- ¾ cup of mayonnaise
- ¼ cup of white wine vinegar, such as Chardonnay
- 1 to 2 tbsp granulated sugar
- 2 tsp celery seeds
- Kosher salt and freshly ground black pepper
- 1 cup of matchstick carrots
- ¼ cup of fresh parsley leaves

Instructions

1. Remove and discard the rough outer leaves of the green cabbage. Cut the head in half, going all the way through the core. Remove the core from both halves with the tip of the knife, then cut each half into quarters. Cut each quarter into small pieces. Repeat with the red cabbage, then combine both in a large mixing bowl.
2. Mix the vinegar, mayonnaise, sugar, and celery seeds in a mini bowl, then season with salt and pepper. As desired, add more sugar. Toss the cabbage with half of the dressing and arrange in a shallow dish (a 9-by-13-inch baking dish works well). Refrigerate for 1 to 2 hours, covered.
3. After the cabbage has marinated in the dressing, taste it and add any remaining dressing as required. Toss in the carrots and parsley to mix.

115. CRANBERRY-ORANGE SALAD

Total Time: 15 Mins

Servings: 8

Ingredients

- quarts ground cranberries
- 2 cups of sugar
- ½ orange, rind of, ground
- 2 peeled oranges
- ¾ cup of walnuts, semi-coarsely chopped
- 3 ½ ounce orange Jell-O

Instructions

1. Grind the cranberries, oranges, rind, and sugar together.
2. Make the Jello with half the amount of water suggested. Stir quickly until completely dissolved.
3. Add nuts to the cranberry mixture.
4. Allow to chill overnight.

116. DIJON MUSTARD VINAIGRETTE

Total Time: 5 Mins

Servings: 1 Cup

Ingredients

- ¼ cup of balsamic vinegar
- 1 tbsp Dijon mustard
- ½ tsp salt
- ¼ tsp coarsely ground pepper
- ¾ cup of extra virgin olive oil

Instructions

1. In a large mixing bowl, combine the first four ingredients. Stirring constantly, slowly add the olive oil.

117. COLE SLAW

Total Time: 20 Mins

Servings: 12

Ingredients

- 6 cups of shredded cabbage
- 1 cup of shredded carrot
- 1 cup of mayonnaise
- ¼ cup of white wine vinegar
- 1 tsp celery seed
- ¼ cup of sugar
- Salt and pepper

Instructions

2. Mix cabbage and carrots in a large mixing bowl. Make the dressing in a smaller bowl by mixing mayonnaise, vinegar, celery seed, sugar, salt, and pepper. Combine the dressing with the cabbage mixture, then put aside to cool. Serve it in a large family-style bowl.

118. EGGPLANT AND TOMATO SAUCE

Prep Time: 5 Mins

Cook Time: 20 Mins

Total Time: 25 Mins

Servings: 4

Ingredients

- 1 medium eggplant (cut in ½ -inch cubes)
- 4 cloves of garlic (smashed and chopped)
- 2 tbsp extra virgin olive oil
- 28-ounce can of plum tomatoes, including juice
- salt and fresh ground pepper
- chopped basil or parsley (for garnish)

Instructions

1. Heat the oil in a big deep skillet over medium-high heat and sauté the garlic in olive oil.
2. Cook for 3 minutes or until the eggplant begins to soften.
3. Chop the tomatoes coarsely and put them to the pan with the juices.
4. Sprinkle with salt and pepper and cook uncovered for 15-20 minutes.
5. Serve with your favorite pasta and fresh herbs.

119. FRENCH DRESSING

Prep Time: 5 Mins

Servings: 3

Ingredients

- 1 tsp Dijon mustard
- 2 tbsp white wine vinegar
- 6 tbsp extra virgin olive oil
- a pinch of sugar

Instructions

1. In a mini bowl, mix together the Dijon mustard, white wine vinegar, extra virgin olive oil, a touch of salt, sugar, and pepper, or mix together in a jam jar.

120. CHUNKY CHICKEN SALAD

Total Time: 10 Mins

Servings: 4

Ingredients

- 1 ½- 2 cups of chicken breasts, cooked and diced into ¾-inch pieces
- ⅛ cup of onion, chopped small
- ⅛ cup of celery, diced small, optional
- 1 tbsp sweet pickle relish
- 3-4 tbsp of mayonnaise
- Paprika
- salt and pepper, to taste

Instructions

1. Combine mayo, onions, relish, and 2 dashes of paprika in a medium bowl.
2. Fold the chicken into the mayonnaise until well mixed.
3. Season with salt and pepper to taste.
4. Chill well before serving over lettuce or over your favorite toast.
5. Note: For this salad, I microwave 2 boneless chicken breast halves sprinkled with salt, pepper, Italian seasoning, garlic powder, and onion powder for 5–6 minutes.
6. If you use leftover chicken, you may need to adjust the seasonings listed in the ingredients.

121. CRANBERRY JELLO SALAD

Total Time: 10 Mins

Servings: 12

Ingredients

- 6 ounces of raspberry jello
- 2 cups of boiling hot water
- 2 cups of cold water
- Two 14 ounce cans whole berry cranberry sauce
- Two 20-ounce cans of crushed pineapple (not pineapple chunks)
- 1 cup of walnuts toasted and chopped

Instructions

1. Using a mixer, combine the 2 (6 ounce) packets of raspberry Jell-O powder and 2 cups of hot water in a big measuring cup. Then mix in 2 cups of cold water until everything is dissolved.
2. Mix the 2 (14 ounce) cans of whole berry cranberry sauce, 2 (20 ounce) cans of crushed pineapple (juice included), and 1 cup of toasted chopped walnuts in a large bowl. Then add the jello and stir until fully combined.
3. Fill a big pan with raised edges or individual cups with the cranberry jello. Refrigerate overnight until it set.

Notes

1. Use crushed pineapple instead of pineapple pieces. The cans seem to be the same, yet they are not. The chunks contain more liquid, resulting in soupy jello.
2. Don't skip toasting the walnuts. It gives the meal a more nutty taste.
3. If you can't locate raspberry jello, you may use cherry, cranberry, or strawberry jello.

122. SMASHED PEA TOAST WITH MARINATED FETA

Prep Time: 20 Mins

Cook Time: 10 Mins

Total Time: 30 Mins

Servings : 20 Crostini

Ingredients

- ⅓ cup of extra-virgin olive oil, with more for brushing the crostini
- ½ cup of feta, preferably sheep's milk
- 1 baguette, cut diagonally into ⅓-inch-thick slices
- 1 tsp of fresh thyme leaves
- ¾ tsp kosher salt, and more for seasoning the crostini
- 1 cup of defrosted, shelled fresh
- freshly ground black pepper
- ¼ tsp red pepper flakes
- Zest and juice of 1 lemon
- 5 mint leaves

Instructions

1. Preheat the oven to 350 degrees Fahrenheit.
2. Put the baguette pieces in a single layer on a rimmed baking sheet. With a pastry brush, brush both sides of each toast with olive oil and sprinkle with salt and pepper. Cook for about 10 minutes until the crostini are crisp but not brown. Remove from the oven. Allow to cool. Crostini are best served the day they are prepared.
3. Crumble the feta into big chunks in a bowl and toss with half of the olive oil, thyme, red pepper flakes, and lemon zest. Let to stand for 30 minutes after gently mixing to blend. (The marinated feta may be made ahead of time; cover firmly and refrigerate for up to 3 days, then bring to room temperature before using.)
4. Heat up a small pot of salted water. Simmer until the peas are just cooked, around 5 minutes. Drain and place in a food processor bowl. Pulse in the remaining olive oil, mint, salt, and lemon juice to make a thick mash.
5. Spread some pea mash on each crostini and sprinkle with marinated feta and freshly crushed black pepper.

123. EASY HONEY MUSTARD RECIPE

Total Time: 5 Mins

Servings: 25

Ingredients

- ⅓ cup of mayonnaise
- ¼ cup of Dijon mustard
- 2 tbsp of yellow mustard
- ¼ cup of honey-plus more to taste
- 1 tbsp white vinegar—or fresh lemon juice or apple cider vinegar
- salt and pepper-to taste
- ½ tsp paprika-optional

Instructions

1. In a small bowl, mix all ingredients. To taste, season with salt and black pepper.
2. Refrigerate in an airtight container for up to 2 weeks.

Notes

1. ¼ tsp cayenne pepper can be added for more heat.
2. Approximately 1 cup of yield.

124. GINGER SALAD DRESSING

Prep Time: 5 Mins

Total Time: 5 Mins

Servings: ¾ Cup

Ingredients

- ½ cup of extra-virgin olive oil
- 2 tbsp of apple cider vinegar to taste
- 2 tbsp Dijon mustard
- 1 tbsp of maple syrup or honey, to taste
- 20 freshly ground black pepper twists
- 2 tsp finely grated fresh ginger
- ½ tsp fine sea salt

Instructions

1. Combine all ingredients in a jar until thoroughly combined. If your mustard is cold, it may take a few minutes to warm up before fully incorporating.
2. Taste and adjust if necessary. If you want more tartness, add another tsp of apple cider vinegar. If you want more sweetness or balance, add another tsp or two of maple syrup (I usually add one).
3. In the refrigerator, this salad dressing can keep for up to 10 days. Real olive oil can get a little solid when it's cold. If this happens, just allow it sit at room temperature for a few minutes or heat it in a microwave-safe jar for 15 to 30 seconds.

125. OLD FASHIONED TURNIP SALAD

Prep Time: 45 Mins

Cook Time: 15 Mins

Total Time: 1 Hour

Servings: 4 Cups

Ingredients

- 5 medium Turnips
- 3 hard-boiled eggs
- 1 cup of chopped celery
- ¼ tsp garlic salt
- ½ cup of chopped onion
- ½ cup of dill pickle relish
- ¼ tsp celery salt
- ground black pepper to taste
- 1 tbsp prepared mustard
- ½ cup of mayonnaise

Instructions

1. Assembly
2. Turnips, eggs, celery, onion, relish, mustard, pepper, mayonnaise, celery salt, and celery are all mixed together in a large bowl. Combine well, then chill in the refrigerator.

For the Stove Top

1. Boiling water with salt in a big saucepan. Cook for 15 minutes, or until turnips are cooked but still firm.
2. Drain, dice, peel, and chop.
3. Add cold water to the pan with the eggs. Bring water to a boil; cover, remove from heat, and set eggs aside for 10 to 12 minutes in boiling water. Remove from the boiling water, allow to cool, then peel and chop.
4. Go to the assembly for the turnip salad.

For the Electric Pressure Cooker (Instant Pot)

5. Remove the tops and tails of your turnips. Then peel your turnips.

6. Cut turnips into cubes and place in a steamer basket.
7. Top the turnip cubes with your eggs.
8. Place the steamer basket into the liner and add 112 cups of water.
9. Put your cooker's lid on and secure it.
10. Turn the vent to sealing and let it run for 4 minutes.
11. Allow the natural pressure to relax for four to five minutes, then quickly release any leftover pressure.
12. Put eggs in an ice bath for 4 minutes until you can handle them.
13. Continue with Turnip Salad assembly.

126. CHINESE CHICKEN SALAD WITH RED CHILE PEANUT DRESSING

Total Time: 20 Mins

Servings: 4

Ingredients

- ¼ cup of rice wine vinegar
- 2 tbsp of smooth peanut butter
- 1 tbsp chopped fresh ginger
- 2 tsp chipotle pepper puree
- 1 tbsp soy sauce
- 1 tbsp honey
- 2 tsp toasted sesame oil
- ½ cup of canola oil
- Salt and freshly ground pepper
- ½ head of Napa cabbage, shredded
- ½ head of romaine lettuce, shredded
- 2 carrots, shredded
- ¼ pound snow peas, julienned
- ¼ cup of coarsely chopped fresh cilantro leaves
- ¼ cup of thinly sliced green onion
- 2 cups of shredded rotisserie chicken
- ½ cup of chopped roasted peanuts
- ¼ cup of chopped fresh mint leaves
- Chili oil, optional

- Grilled lime halves for garnish

Instructions

1. Mix the vinegar, peanut butter, ginger, soy sauce, honey, sesame oil, and canola in a medium bowl. Mix salt and pepper, if desired, to taste. In a large bowl, mix the cabbage, lettuce, carrots, snow peas, cilantro, and green onion. Toss to mix after adding the dressing.
2. Add the chicken, chopped peanuts, and mint on the serving dish before transfer. If desired, drizzle with chili oil. Grilled lime halves are a garnish.

127. EASY LIME VINAIGRETTE

Total Time: 5 Mins

Servings: ½ Cup

Ingredients

- ¼ tsp kosher salt, plus more if needed
- 1 lime: 1 tbsp of lime zest and 2 tbsp of lime juice
- ½ cup of olive oil
- ½ tsp maple syrup
- ½ tbsp Dijon mustard

Instructions

1. lime; zest it. Sprinkle with kosher salt and cut as finely as possible. Holding the knife's dull edge, scrape the sharp edge over the chopped lime zest while angling the blade to combine the zest into a paste. Take your time with this; it should only take a minute or two to complete.
2. Mix the Dijon mustard, lime juice, and maple syrup with the zest in a medium bowl. 1 tbsp at a time (8 total tbsp) at first, mix in the olive oil until smooth and emulsified. Season with extra salt if required.

128. WALDORF SALAD RECIPE

Total Time: 15 Mins

Servings: 2

Ingredients

- 2 Granny Smith apples
- 1 cup of salted shelled walnuts
- 1 cup of chopped celery
- 1 cup of seedless green grapes
- ½ cup of mayonnaise
- ½ tsp kosher salt
- 4 iceberg lettuce leaves for the bowl's garnish
- 1 tbsp of lemon juice

Instructions

1. To make bite-sized pieces, core, and cut apples. Cut the shelled walnuts roughly. To a bowl, add both.
2. Add green grapes and sliced celery (you can halve them if you prefer).
3. Mix mayonnaise, salt, and lemon juice in a small bowl. Place on the apple mixture.
4. Before serving, use iceberg lettuce leaves to cover a bowl (or two separate bowls). Serve salad in bowls. Enjoy!

Notes

1. Apple Waldorf salad is best eaten the same day it is prepared, but it may be refrigerated for 3 days.
2. Change: Change the green grapes with red grapes. Instead of walnuts, use pecans. For a bit more taste, sprinkle some black pepper on top!

129. LEMON DRESSING

Total Time: 5 Mins

Servings: ½ Cup

Ingredients

- 1 tsp finely grated lemon zest
- 1 tbsp honey
- ½ tsp chopped thyme
- ¼ cup of extra-virgin olive oil
- Kosher salt and freshly ground pepper

Instructions

1. Mix the lemon juice, honey, and thyme together in a small bowl. Pepper and salt are mixed in after the olive oil.

130. BRIGHT SPRING SALAD

Prep Time: 20 Mins

Cook Time: 1 Mins

Total Time: 21 Mins

Servings: 4

Ingredients

- 1 bunch of asparagus, tender parts, chopped into 1-inch pieces
- ½ cup of thawed frozen peas
- A few handfuls of salad greens
- 2 thinly sliced radishes
- ½ cup of crumbled feta cheese
- ½ pitted and diced avocado
- ¼ cup of chopped, toasted pistachios
- Sea salt and freshly ground pepper
- ½ cup of roasted chickpeas
- Fresh herbs for garnish (basil, mint, or chives)

Dressing

- ¼ cup of fresh basil
- 1 small garlic clove
- 1 tbsp white wine vinegar
- 1 tbsp lemon juice, plus ½ tsp zest
- 2 tbsp of extra-virgin olive oil, more as desired
- ¼ tsp sea salt

Instructions

1. Set a bowl of cold water nearby and bring a big pot of salted water to a boil. Blanch the asparagus for about 1 minute, or until tender but still brilliant green. Transfer for one minute to the ice water, then drain. Let the asparagus dry, put it back in the bowl, and then add the peas.
2. To prepare the dressing: Pulse the herbs, garlic, lemon juice, lemon zest, vinegar, olive oil, and salt in a food processor to combine.
3. Toss the asparagus with the remaining half of the dressing in a bowl. Use salt and pepper to taste to season.
4. assemble the salad. Layer the salad greens, asparagus/pea combination, radishes, feta, avocado, pistachios, chickpeas, and herbs on a plate. Serve with the remaining dressing and more salt and pepper to taste.

131. CRISPY CHICKEN SALAD WITH HONEY MUSTARD DRESSING

Prep Time: 20 Mins

Cook Time: 20 Mins

Total Time: 40 Mins

Servings: 6

Ingredients

- 2 tbsp of raw honey melted
- ¼ cup of stone ground mustard
- 1 ½ tbsp of fresh lemon juice
- 3 tbsp of olive oil
- sea salt and black pepper to taste
- 1 pound of sliced, boneless, skinless chicken breasts
- ¾ cup of blanched almond flour
- ¼ cup of arrowroot flour or tapioca
- ¾ tsp sea salt
- ¼ tsp freshly ground black pepper
- 1 large egg whisked
- 3-4 tbsp of refined coconut oil or avocado
- 4-6 slices of nitrate-free bacon, cooked and crumbled
- 1 medium avocado sliced
- 4 large eggs hardboiled and sliced
- ¾ cup of cherry tomatoes halved
- 5-ounce container salad greens or the equivalent fresh greens

Instructions

Dressing

1. I prefer to have this ready first. For the version with honey, mix all ingredients in a bowl except the oil with a mixer, and then gently add the oil while still stirring.
2. In a high-speed mixer or food processor, combine the ingredients for the Whole30 version and mix until completely smooth. Add the oil in a gentle stream while the mixer is still running until everything is combined. Add salt and pepper to taste and season.

For the Salad

3. Before preparing the chicken, have the bacon and eggs cooked, crumbled, sliced, and prepared.
4. In a mini bowl, combine the arrowroot and almond flour with the salt and pepper. mix the egg and one tsp of water in a separate shallow bowl. Add a little amount of more sea salt and pepper to the chicken.
5. Heat the oil in a large skillet over medium-high heat. Once the oil is heated enough, dip a piece of chicken in the egg, brushing off excess, then coat with the dry mixture and place in the skillet. Continue by using all the chicken pieces.
6. Cook for about 3 minutes, turning the food frequently until the surface is golden brown. Turn gently with tongs so that the breading does not fall off. Depending on thickness, cook for 5 minutes on the second side until golden brown and well done.
7. Put the chicken on a cutting board and let it cool for a few minutes. Then, cut it into small pieces.
8. Assemble the salad by placing the greens, bacon, sliced eggs, tomatoes, avocado, and chicken in a large serving bowl. Serve right away with a drizzle of dressing or with a side of dressing for dipping. Drizzle with dressing. Enjoy!
9. Notes
10. Use ¼ cup of packed, pitted, softened Medjool dates and 2 ½ tsp water for the Whole30 version.
11. Arrange it on a baking sheet coated with parchment paper and bake for 15 to 18 minutes, depending on the type of bacon and your preference. On paper towels, drain.
12. Put the eggs in a medium saucepan, cover with water, and bring to a boil. This is how I hard boil eggs. Cut the heat off and cover. After 13 to 15 minutes of steaming in the covered pot, take the eggs and chill them in a bowl of ice water before peeling.

132. TAPENADE

Total Time: 10 Mins

Prep Time: 10 Mins

Servings: ½ Cups

Ingredients

- ½ pound of pitted mixed olives
- 2 anchovy fillets, rinsed
- 1 small minced garlic clove
- 2 tbsp capers
- 2 to 3 fresh basil leaves
- 1 tbsp freshly squeezed lemon juice
- 2 tbsp extra-virgin olive oil

Instructions

1. In cold water, thoroughly rinse the olives. Combine ingredients in a food processor. Process until the mixture produces a coarse paste, about 1 to 2 minutes total, stopping to scrape down the sides of the bowl. Place in a bowl, then serve.

133. MISO GLAZED COD WITH SAUTEED SPINACH & ONIONS

Prep Time: 10 Mins

Cook Time: 25 Mins

Total Time: 35 Mins

Servings: 4

Ingredients

For the Sauteed Spinach and Onions

- 2 tbsp oil
- 1 red onion
- ½ tsp fresh grated ginger
- 2 cups of frozen spinach
- 2 tsp soy sauce or Tamari
- 1 tsp white sesame and 1 tsp black sesame
- Chili flakes to garnish

For the Miso Glazed Cod

- 1 pound of cod
- 2 tbsp of oil (to coat bottom of the pan)
- 2 tbsp white miso
- 2 tbsp honey
- 1 tbsp soy sauce or Tamari
- 1 tsp of fresh grated ginger
- 1 tbsp chili flakes

Instructions

1. Peel and slice the onion first (I chopped it so there were long thin pieces).
2. Using a microplane grater, peel and grate a knob of ginger to make 12 tsp (for the spinach) and 1 tsp (for the cod) of freshly grated ginger.
3. Set a pan over medium heat with a layer of oil on the bottom.
4. Cook for 5 minutes after adding the onion.
5. Then add the ginger and cook for 5 minutes more.
6. Add the frozen spinach and cook it until it is heated through (about 5 more minutes or so).

7. Then toss in the soy sauce and sesame seeds until fully combined.
8. Take it from the pan and place it in a basin. Set aside, covered, until the cod is done.
9. Let's make the miso glaze by mixing the white miso, honey, soy sauce, and ginger together very well.
10. Then stir in the chile flakes until completely combined.
11. Rinse and wipe dry the fish before slicing it into individual servings.
12. Then brush the miso glaze on one side of the fish pieces.
13. Add around 1 tbsp of oil to the same saucepan you used to cook the spinach and delicately swirl it around the bottom of the pan.
14. Add the cod, miso-glazed side down, and simmer for approximately 4-5 minutes, or until the miso glaze caramelizes and the cod is done.
15. Turn the fish over and simmer the other side after brushing the miso glaze on the opposite side. Cook for 3-4 minutes more, or until the fish flakes easily when prodded with a fork.
16. Warm cod with spinach and onions.

134. CLASSIC POTATO SALAD RECIPE

Prep Time: 10 Mins

Cook Time: 20 Mins

Chilling Time: 1 Hr 30 Mins

Total Time: 2 Hrs

Servings: 12

Ingredients

- 4 pounds of peeled and cubed ¾ -inch-thick russet potatoes
- Kosher salt
- ¼ cup of divided sugar
- 6 tbsp divided rice wine vinegar
- 3 ribs of finely diced celery
- 1 medium finely chopped red onion
- 4 scallions, green parts only, thinly sliced, optional
- ¼ cup of fresh parsley leaves washed and minced (optional)
- ¼ cup of chopped cornichons
- 2 tbsp of whole grain mustard (more or less to taste)
- 1 ¼ cups of mayonnaise

- Fresh ground black pepper

Instructions

1. To a large saucepan, add 2 quarts of water. Add 2 tsp each of kosher salt, sugar, and vinegar, along with the potatoes. Using high heat, bring to a boil. Reduce the heat to a simmer and boil the potatoes for about 10 minutes, stirring occasionally. Transfer potatoes to a baking sheet with a rim. Sprinkle 2 tsp of vinegar over the evenly distributed layer. Allow to cool for around 30 minutes till room temperature.
2. Mix remaining sugar, remaining vinegar, celery, onion, scallion, parsley, pickles, mustard, and mayonnaise in a big bowl. To combine, stir with a rubber spatula. Stir in the potatoes. Use salt and pepper to taste to season. Refrigerate for at least one hour and up to three days before serving.

135. ASIAN SESAME DRESSING

Total Time: 3 Mins

Servings: 1 Cup

Ingredients

Big batch to keep (makes 1 cup)

- ¼ cup of soy sauce
- 2 tbsp toasted sesame oil
- ¼ cup of white vinegar (adjust to taste for sharpness)
- ¼ cup of olive oil
- 1 tbsp sugar (any type) or 1 ½ tbsp honey

Single serving batch

- 1 tbsp soy sauce
- 2 tsp toasted sesame oil
- 1 tbsp white vinegar
- 1 tbsp olive oil (Note 1)
- 1 tsp sugar (any type) or 1 ½ tsp honey

Instructions

1. Shake the ingredients in a container until the sugar is dissolved. To taste, add salt to taste for saltiness and sugar for sweetness.
2. Keep in the refrigerator for up to 3 weeks (to be safe). Shake thoroughly and bring to room temp before using.
3. For a side salad for four people, a single serving batch makes enough for 3 to 4 cups of shredded cabbage or other greens.
4. Large batch - my basic rule of thumb for how much dressing to use is 1 tbsp every 1 packed cup of shredded veggies and 2 tsp each handful of leafy greens.

Notes

1. In this dressing, I believe the olive oil is great. You can even use extra-virgin olive oil to make it taste even better. Or otherwise, use any oil with a neutral flavor, such canola, grapeseed, or vegetable oil.

136. WATERCRESS SALAD

Prep Time: 20 Mins

Cook Time: 2 Mins

Total Time: 22 Mins

Servings: 4

Ingredients

- 4 ounces of snap peas
- 1 fennel bulb, cut on a mandoline to a very thin piece
- Champagne Vinaigrette
- 3 cups of watercress
- Segments from ½ navel orange
- 1 sliced ripe avocado,
- 2 ounces of torn fresh mozzarella
- 2 tbsp toasted pistachios
- Sea salt and freshly ground black pepper
- Lemon wedge, for serving

Instructions

2. Set aside a bowl of cold water and bring a large saucepan of salted water to a boil. To blanch the snap peas, place it in the boiling water for 2 minutes. Remove the sugar snap peas and immerse them in the ice water for approximately 15 seconds, or until they are completely cooled. Strain and let it dry on a kitchen towel or some paper towels.
3. Mix the sliced fennel with 1 to 2 tbsp of the dressing and a sprinkle of salt in a small bowl. To coat, toss gently.
4. Put the watercress, fennel, snap peas, orange segments, avocado, and mozzarella on a dish and assemble the salad. Add the pistachios and drizzle some of the dressing on top. Sprinkle with salt, pepper, and a squeeze of lemon to taste, and serve.

137. CRISPY KALE SALAD WITH HOMMUS DRESSING

Prep Time: 15 Mins

Cook Time: 50 Mins

Total Time: 1 Hr 5 Mins

Servings: 4

Ingredients

Salad

- 1 chopped and peeled sweet potato
- 2 tbsp olive oil divided
- salt sea salt, to taste
- 3 cups of chopped kale
- 3 tbsp cashews roasted
- 1 tsp chili flakes
- 1 tbsp olive oil extra virgin

Salad Dressing

- ½ cup of hommus
- 1 tsp Dijon mustard
- 1 tbsp lemon juice
- 1 tsp maple syrup

Instructions

Salad

1. Preheat the oven to 200 degrees Celsius.
2. Sweet potato, peeled and sliced into 2cm chunks. Add 1 tbsp of olive oil and season with sea salt.
3. Place the chopped sweet potato on a lined sheet tray. Spread them out without overlap in a single layer.
4. Roast sweet potato for 30 minutes, or until golden brown with crispy pieces on the side. You might want to flip them over halfway through so that both sides get good caramelization.
5. Remove from the oven and set aside to cool.
6. After you've roasted the sweet potatoes, keep the oven at 200°C.
7. Thoroughly wash and dry the kale leaves.
8. Remove the kale stems by making a V-shaped slice along the stems with a sharp knife. Tear up the larger leaves into smaller bits.
9. Massage the kale leaves completely with 1 tbsp of olive oil. Then season with sea salt.
10. Place on a prepared sheet tray and bake for 15 minutes, or until crisp but the leaves are mostly green. Remove from the oven and set aside for a few minutes to cool.

Salad Dressing

11. In a small bowl, combine the hummus, Dijon mustard, lemon juice, and maple syrup.
12. Mix until thoroughly combined.
13. Assembly
14. Spread the hommus dressing in a circular across a serving platter.
15. On one-third of the platter, place crispy kale over hommus dressing, followed by roasted sweet potato.
16. Crush the roasted cashews into smaller pieces and put them over the salad.
17. Finished with an extra virgin olive oil drizzling and a sprinkle of chili flakes.
18. Serve.

Notes

1. Crispy kale is a tasty snack, so prepare a double batch to save for later. It is best consumed within a few hours.
2. You may use roasted pumpkin for the sweet potato in this recipe.
3. To make a nut-free version, use pepitas instead of cashew nuts.

138. BABY BOK CHOY SALAD WITH SESAME DRESSING

Prep Time: 5 Mins

Cook Time: 25 Mins

Total Time: 30 Mins

Servings: 8

Ingredients

For the sesame dressing

- ¼ cup of light brown sugar
- ¼ cup of olive oil
- 2 tbsp red wine vinegar
- 2 tbsp toasted sesame seeds (see notes)
- 1 tbsp soy sauce

For the salad

- 2 tbsp olive oil
- 1 package of ramen noodles crumbled, seasoning packet discarded (see notes for vegan information)
- ¼ cup of sliced almonds
- 1 bunch baby bok choy sliced (5 – 6 bulbs)
- 5 chopped scallions

Instructions

1. To make the dressing, mix together brown sugar, olive oil, vinegar, sesame seeds, and soy sauce in a small bowl. While making the rest of the salad, let the flavors to mix at room temperature.
2. Heat the olive oil in a large saucepan over medium heat until it shimmers. Turn the heat down low. Sauté the ramen noodles and almonds for about 10 minutes, often stirring to avoid scorching.
3. Combine the baby bok choy, scallions, and crunchy mix in a large bowl. Toss the salad with the salad dressing until evenly combined. At room temperature, serve.

Notes

1. You may buy toasted sesame seeds or roast normal sesame seeds at home.
2. Heat the sesame seeds in a medium pan over medium heat until golden brown and aromatic, about 3-5 minutes, stirring occasionally.
3. Remove from the fire and place on a plate to cool entirely. Store in a pantry airtight container for 6 months or in a freezer storage bag for up to 1 year.
4. to prepare ahead of time
5. Combine Sesame Dressing ingredients and refrigerate covered.
6. The baby bok choy and scallions can be cut and refrigerated separately in separate containers.
7. Toasted, cooled, and kept at room temperature, the crunchy mix may be made ahead of time.
8. I suggest preparing the ingredients no more than one day ahead of time.
9. To make the salad gluten-free:
10. Remove the ramen noodles.
11. Substitute gluten-free soy sauce
12. To make the salad vegan:
13. Choose Top Ramen brand ramen noodles that are completely vegan.

139. ICEBERG LETTUCE SALAD

Total Time: 10 Mins

Servings: 4

Ingredients

- ¼ large iceberg lettuce head, shredded
- 3 small sliced cucumbers
- 4 small sliced Campari tomatoes
- 6 medium sliced radishes
- 1 medium sliced bell pepper
- ¼ cup of chopped fresh dill
- ¼ cup of hemp seeds
- 1 tbsp apple cider vinegar
- 2 tbsp olive oil
- ¾ tsp sea salt or to taste
- ¼ tsp pepper or to taste

Instructions

1. In a large bowl, combine the veggies, dill, and hemp seeds.
2. Combine the olive oil, apple cider vinegar, salt, and pepper in a mixing bowl. Serve right away.

Notes

1. Add other vegetables. You can add any vegetables you like to this salad, such as carrots, broccoli, beets, onions, and more. Just chop them to the same size as the other vegetables in the salad.
2. Replace the dressing with another. Feel free to try other delicious vegan dressings on this great salad. It's so versatile that it could go with a balsamic, ranch, Italian, or Russian dressing.
3. Add protein. By adding protein, you can make this Iceberg Lettuce Salad more filling. Try black beans, tofu cubes, or green lentils.
4. Mix in the fruits and nuts. This recipe would be great with apples, pears, and cranberries. You may also add in some chopped almonds, walnuts, or cashews.

140. MARINATED MUSHROOM SALAD IN ITALIAN DRESSING

Prep Time: 5 Mins

Cook Time: 8 Mins

Total Time: 13 Mins

Servings: 6

Ingredients

- 24-ounce fresh white button mushrooms
- 1 tbsp vinegar
- 2 pinches of salt
- 4 crushed garlic cloves
- 3 tbsp chopped green onions
- ½ cup of Italian Dressing Wishbone

Instructions

1. Boil a pot of water (a little more than halfway full). When the water has reached a boil, add some salt, 1 tbsp vinegar, and the mushrooms.

2. Boil for 10 minutes from the time you throw them into the water.
3. Before adding any other ingredients, drain and let cool completely.
4. When the mushrooms have cooled, mix them with ½ cup of Italian dressing, 3 tbsp chopped green onions and 4 cloves of crushed garlic.
5. Refrigerate for 6 hours or overnight. Serve salad cold.

141. PINEAPPLE-PECAN CHICKEN SALAD

Total Time: 20 Mins

Servings: 6

Ingredients

- 3 cup of chopped cooked chicken breasts
- 1 cup of finely chopped celery
- 2 sliced green onions
- 2 tbsp finely chopped green pepper
- 1 tsp salt
- dash of black pepper
- ½ cup of mayonnaise
- ½ cup of chopped pecans
- 20-ounce drained pineapple tidbits
- 2 tbsp lemon juice

Instructions

1. Mix the chicken, celery, green onion, green pepper, salt, black pepper, and mayonnaise in a bowl.
2. Mix in the pecans, pineapple, and lemon juice.
3. Allow flavors to mix for about 30 minutes before serving.

142. BRAISED ARTICHOKES, TOMATO & THYME LINGUINE

Total Time: 1 Hr

Servings: 4

Ingredients

- 1 lemon
- 4 medium artichokes
- 2 tbsp olive oil
- 1 sliced onion
- 3 crushed garlic cloves
- 2 ripe tomatoes, peeled and chopped
- 1 tbsp chopped fresh thyme leaves
- 2 cups of chicken stock or water
- salt and pepper
- 375g linguine or long, thin pasta
- freshly grated parmesan, to serve

Instructions

1. **To prepare the artichoke:** Squeeze the juice from half a lemon into a large bowl of cold water. Fill the bowl with the lemon halves.
2. Working with one artichoke at a time, put it in the water bath if it starts to turn brown as you work.
3. Bend back and snap off the rough outer leaves of the artichoke to begin the real preparation. Remove many layers of leaves until you have mostly pale green or yellow leaves with yellow tips. Cut the dark green, pointed leaf tips. (Cut about 1 inch from a medium artichoke.)
4. Trim the stem's base and peel away the dark green outer layer of skin using a vegetable peeler. Using a knife, remove any dark green leaf bases that remain around the stem's top.
5. The artichoke is then quartered lengthwise, with a part of the each piece has a stem connected. Starting at the stem end of each quarter, slide a tiny, sharp knife under the fuzzy choke and cut toward the leaf tips. Take out the choke.

6. Clean the artichoke quarters and cut them into ¼ inch thick slices. Place the wedges in the bowl of acidulated water. Repeat the procedure with the next artichoke once the first has been entirely trimmed.

7. Cook onion and garlic in oil in a deep frying pan over medium heat for 4-5 minutes, or until softened and fragrant. Cook for 5 minutes, occasionally stirring, with the tomatoes.

8. Season with salt and add the drained artichokes, thyme, and stock. Cook for 20-30 minutes, or until the sauce has reduced and the artichokes are soft.

9. Cook pasta until cooked in boiling salted water; drain and mix with sauce. Season with salt and pepper to taste and divide into four serving bowls. Serve immediately topped with parmesan.

143. CARAMELIZED LEEKS OVER NOODLES

Total Time: 55 Mins

Servings: 2

Ingredients

- 2 medium leeks
- ½ tbsp olive oil
- 1 tbsp butter
- ½ tbsp dark brown sugar
- 5 ounces of egg noodles
- 2 tbsp chopped fresh parsley
- 1 tsp extra virgin olive oil
- salt and black pepper

Instructions

1. Split the leeks lengthwise and gently wash each layer.
2. Cut across into thin strips, including the green part.
3. Gently heat the oil and butter together.
4. When the butter has melted, mix in the leeks.
5. Cook, uncovered, for approximately 10 minutes, or until the leeks soften.
6. Sprinkle the sugar on top, and after a couple more minutes, mix well.
7. Cook for another 15-30 minutes until the leeks have collapsed into a sticky mass.
8. If necessary, add small amounts of hot water to prevent sticking.
9. Cook and rinse the noodles while the leeks are cooking.

10. When the leeks are done, add the parsley, olive oil, cooked noodles, and salt to taste.
11. Toss thoroughly and serve.

144. OVEN BAKED CHICKEN BREAST WITH PESTO, MOZZARELLA AND WRAPPED IN BACON

Prep Time: 5 Mins

Cook Time: 35 Mins

Total Time: 40 Mins

Servings: 4

Ingredients

- 4 chicken breasts
- 4 tsp pesto
- 5-ounce Mozzarella divided into four pieces
- 8 slices bacon
- 4 tbsp breadcrumbs
- 5 sun-dried tomatoes
- 4 tbsp Parmesan Grated

Instructions

1. Preheat the oven to 430 degrees Fahrenheit.
2. Using a knife, cut the chicken about ¾ vertically. Not entirely, but leave the back of the chicken attached, so you have an envelope.
3. 4 breasts of chicken
4. Put pesto on the inside and stuff a slice of Mozzarella into the pocket. Then close it.
5. 4 tsp pesto, 5 ounces mozzarella
6. 2 pieces of bacon wrapped around the chicken
7. 8 bacon slices
8. Place the chicken in a baking sheet and repeat the first four steps with the other chicken breasts.
9. Spread the sun-dried tomatoes on top of the chicken breasts.
10. 5 dried sun-dried tomatoes
11. Garnish with breadcrumbs and Parmesan cheese.
12. 4 tbsp breadcrumbs, 4 tbsp Parmesan cheese

13. Cook the chicken for 35 minutes or until done. Serve right away.

Notes

1. **Pesto -** a smooth sauce made with pine nuts, olive oil, basil, salt, Parmesan cheese, and garlic. It has a lot of flavors, and it goes well with chicken. It can be substituted with red (Sicilian) pesto or tapenade.
2. **Chicken breast -** Use boneless chicken breast.
3. **Substitutes -** Parmesan Cheese - I The flavor of this hard Italian cheese is salty, nutty, and spicy. It's amazing to add extra flavor when grated on top of a dish. It can be replaced with Grana Padano (which is a bit milder).
4. **Serve with -** Pasta Cooked (spaghetti, Penne, and Fusilli are great choices). Combine with a green salad, such as this strawberry, arugula, and pistachio salad, or this tomato salad with Parmesan, pesto, and pine nuts.

145. CHICKEN CACCIATORE

Prep Time: 10 Mins

Cook Time: 40 Mins

Total Time: 50 Mins

Servings: 6

Ingredients

- 3 tbsp divided olive oil
- 6 bone-in skinless chicken thighs
- Salt and pepper to season
- 1 medium diced onion
- 2 tbsp minced garlic
- 1 small diced yellow bell pepper (capsicum)
- 1 small diced red bell pepper (capsicum)
- 1 large peeled and sliced carrot
- 10-ounce sliced mushrooms
- ½ cup of pitted black olives
- 8 sprigs thyme
- 1 tsp dried oregano
- 2 tbsp each freshly cut parsley and basil plus more to garnish

- 150ml red wine
- 28-ounce crushed tomatoes
- 2 tbsp tomato paste
- 7-ounce halved Roma tomatoes
- ½ tsp red pepper flakes

Instructions

1. Add salt and pepper to taste to the chicken.
2. In a big cast iron skillet, heat 2 tbsp of oil. Cook the chicken over high heat until brown on both sides, about 3–4 minutes on each side. Remove from skillet and put aside.
3. Pour in the remaining oil into the pan. Simmer until the onion is transparent, about 3-4 minutes. Cook for 30 seconds, or until the garlic is fragrant. Cook for 5 minutes until the peppers, carrots, mushrooms, and herbs begin to soften.
4. Pour the wine, scraping off any browned bits from the bottom of the skillet. Cook for 2 minutes, or until the wine has reduced.
5. Combine crushed tomatoes, tomato paste, Roma tomatoes, and chili flakes in a mixing bowl. Season to taste with salt and pepper. Transfer the chicken pieces to the skillet and cook on the stovetop.
6. **For stove top**
7. Combine all of the ingredients; cover with a lid, lower to low heat, and leave to simmer for 40 minutes, or until the meat comes from the bone. Allow the olives to boil for another 10 minutes. Garnish with parsley and serve right away.
8. **For the oven**
9. Cook the covered skillet in a preheated oven at 375°F for 50 minutes. Remove the top and cook for another 20 minutes, or until the chicken is cooked and falling off the bone and the sauce has reduced.

Notes

1. Use this recipe in the slow cooker.
2. If the sauce is too thin for you, thicken it with 2 tbsp more tomato paste while it's simmering.
3. **To Prepare Ahead:** Cool, cover, and refrigerate this chicken cacciatore up to 1 day ahead of time. Reheat on low-medium heat.
4. **To freeze:** Place the cooled cacciatore in an airtight container and place in the freezer. Thaw it out in the morning before serving and bring to room temperature. Transfer to a skillet or pan and cook over low-medium heat until well warmed..

146. CHICKEN WITH FORTY CLOVES OF GARLIC

Total Time: 1 Hr 40 Mins

Prep Time: 35 Mins

Cook Time: 1 Hr 15 Mins

Servings: 6

Ingredients

- 3 whole heads of garlic
- 3 ½ -pound chickens, cut into eighths
- Kosher salt
- Freshly ground black pepper
- 1 tbsp unsalted butter
- 2 tbsp good olive oil
- 3 tbsp Cognac, divided
- 1 ½ cups of dry white wine
- 1 tbsp fresh thyme leaves
- 2 tbsp all-purpose flour
- 2 tbsp heavy cream

Instructions

1. Separate the garlic cloves and place them in a saucepan of boiling water for 60 seconds. Drain and peel the garlic. Place aside.
2. With paper towels, pat the chicken dry. Sprinkle both sides liberally with salt and pepper. Heat the butter and oil over medium-high heat in a large pot or Dutch oven. Cook the chicken in batches in the fat, skin side down, until well browned, approximately 3 to 5 minutes on each side. You don't want to stick a fork through the skin, so use tongs or a spatula to turn the meat. Reduce the heat to medium if the fat is burning. When one batch of chicken is cooked, transfer it to a platter and continue cooking the other chicken in batches. Transfer the last chicken to a platter and add the remaining garlic to the saucepan. Reduce the heat to low and cook for 5 to 10 minutes, constantly stirring, until evenly browned. Transfer to a boil and scrape the brown pieces from the pan with 2 tbsp of Cognac and wine. Return the chicken to the saucepan with the juices and the thyme leaves. Cover and cook for approximately 30 minutes until the chicken is cooked.

3. Transfer the chicken to a plate and cover with foil to keep warm. Stir together ½ cup of the sauce with the flour in a small bowl, then mix it back into the sauce in the saucepan. Raise the heat to high, add the remaining tbsp of Cognac, and boil for 3 minutes. Season with salt and pepper to taste; it should be quite tasty because chicken is famously bland. Serve the chicken with the sauce and garlic on the side.

147. CLASSIC PESTO RECIPE

Total Time: 10 Mins

Servings: 16 Tbsp

Ingredients

- 4 cups of basil
- 2-3 cloves of garlic
- ¼ cup of pine nuts
- ¾ cup of grated Parmesan cheese
- ½ tsp kosher salt
- ¾ - 1 cup of olive oil

Instructions

1. Mix the basil, garlic, pine nuts, parmesan cheese, and salt in a food processor.
2. Begin the food processor and gently pour olive oil through the chute, stopping to scrape down the edges of the bowl.
3. Refrigerate for a few days, freeze in ice cube trays, and store in zip-top bags for a few months.

Notes

1. Refrigerate pesto in an airtight jar for up to 1 week.
2. Freezer Compatible
3. Place pesto in an ice tray and freeze for 30 minutes. Frozen pesto cubes can be stored for up to a year in a zip-top freezer bag or other airtight, freezer-safe container.

148. BASIL WALNUT PESTO

Total Time: 5 Mins

Servings: 1 Cup

Ingredients

- 2 cups of firmly packed basil
- ½ cup of extra virgin olive oil
- 3 garlic cloves (omit for low-FODMAP)
- ⅓ cup of chopped walnuts
- ⅓ cup of shredded parmesan cheese
- ½ tsp sea salt
- ¼ tsp cracked black pepper
- ¼ tsp red pepper flakes
- zest of 1 lemon plus 1 tsp of lemon juice

Instructions

1. In a food processor fitted with the blade attachment, combine all ingredients except the olive oil. 1 minute, or until the ingredients are mostly broken down and gravelly.
2. Drizzle in the olive oil in a steady stream while the food processor is running, pulsing until combined, and the desired smoothness is obtained.

149. THE BEST BASIC PESTO

Total Time: 15 Mins

Servings: 1 ¼ Cup

Ingredients

- ⅓ cup of walnuts
- 2 large roughly chopped garlic cloves
- 2 cups of gently packed fresh basil leaves
- ½ tsp salt
- ¼ tsp ground black pepper
- ⅔ cup of extra virgin olive oil
- ½ cup of grated Parmigiano-Reggiano

Instructions

1. Mix the walnuts and garlic in the bowl of a food processor fitted with a steel blade. Process for 10 seconds, or until roughly chopped. Process the basil leaves, salt, and pepper until the mixture resembles a paste, approximately 1 minute. Slowly pour the olive oil through the feed tube while the processor is running, and process until the pesto is thoroughly mixed. Add the Parmesan and process for one more minute. Use pesto right away or keep in a carefully sealed jar or airtight plastic container with a thin coating of olive oil on top (this seals out the air and prevents the pesto from oxidizing, which would turn it an ugly brown color). It will last approximately a week in the refrigerator.

150. PARSLEY PESTO

Total Time: 20 Mins

Servings: 10

Ingredients

- ¾ cup of walnuts, pecans, or pine nuts
- 1 cup of chopped parsley, tightly packed
- ½ cup of finely grated pecorino or Parmigiano cheese
- ½ cup of extra virgin olive oil
- ½ tsp salt
- 1 to 2 chopped garlic cloves
- Black pepper to taste

Instructions

2. In a large mortar, combine all of the ingredients except the oil and grind to a firm paste. Drizzle in approximately a quarter of the olive oil and grind it into the pesto until everything is pretty well ground. Repeat with another quarter of the oil, and so on, until all of the oil is mixed into the pesto.
3. Alternatively, place everything except the oil in the bowl of a food processor. While slowly drizzling in the oil, buzz the mixture. The more oil you add, the more like a sauce your pesto will be and less like a condiment.
4. Taste for salt and add more if necessary as the pesto comes together. Serve your parsley pesto immediately, or store it in a covered jar with plastic wrap right on top to keep air out. This helps the color stay bright and nice. Use within a few days.

Notes

1. If you choose to take an additional step, keep the parsley on the stalk and dip it in boiling salted water for 30 seconds, then shock it in freezing water. This sets the color and keeps your pesto green for much longer.

151. SUN-DRIED TOMATO AND WALNUT PESTO

Total Total: 10 Mins

Servings: 2 Cup

Ingredients

- 1 cup of oil-packed sun-dried tomatoes, plus 3 tbsp of oil
- ½ cup of lightly toasted walnuts
- ¼ cup of grated Parmigiano-Reggiano
- ¼ tsp crushed red pepper
- 1 clove of garlic
- ¼ cup of fresh basil leaves
- Salt and freshly ground black pepper

Instructions

2. In a food processor, combine the sun-dried tomatoes with oil, walnuts, cheese, crushed red pepper, and garlic, and process until smooth. Add in the basil and pulse 5 times to keep the color of the herb. Season to taste.

152. BASIL AND WALNUT PESTO

Total Time: 10 Mins

Servings: 12

Ingredients

- 4 cups of basil leaves
- 3 peeled garlic cloves
- ½ cup of walnuts toasted
- ½ cup of parmesan-reggiano
- zest and juice of one lemon
- ¼ tsp red pepper flakes
- ½ cup of extra virgin olive oil, more as needed
- ½ tsp freshly cracked black pepper
- ½ tsp kosher salt

Instructions

1. Add basil, garlic, walnuts, parmesan, lemon zest, juice, and red pepper flakes to the bowl of a food processor.
2. To break down the basil, pulse a few times.
3. Add olive oil in a steady stream, pulsing until it is incorporated with the other ingredients and the mixture forms a loose paste. If your pesto is too thick, add one spoonful of olive oil at a time until it reaches the desired consistency.
4. Season with salt and pepper to taste.
5. Enjoy!

153. RICE NOODLES WITH VEGETABLES

Total Time: 45 Mins

Servings: 4

Ingredients

- 2 medium heads of broccoli sliced into bite-sized florets, or 1 pound of broccoli florets
- 12 to 16 ounces of sliced mushrooms (any variety)
- 2 tbsp of olive oil or sunflower oil

2 tbsp toasted sesame oil

- 1-inch piece of ginger, grated (optional)
- 2 tsp of lime juice (optional)
- Salt

Rice noodles & stir-fry sauce

- 8 ounces of rice noodles (also called stir-fry or pad thai noodles)
- 3 tbsp lower-sodium soy sauce
- 1 tbsp toasted sesame oil
- 1 tbsp plus 1 tsp maple syrup
- 1 ½ tsp balsamic vinegar
- 1 garlic clove, finely chopped or grated

Instructions

1. Preheat the oven to 450 degrees Fahrenheit.
2. Spread the broccoli and mushrooms on 3 baking sheets and drizzle them with sesame oil and olive oil. To coat the veggies evenly, toss them with your hands. If the veggies appear to be dry, add a little extra oil.
3. Toss the vegetables again with the ginger (optional). Spread the vegetables on the baking sheets in a single layer, evenly spaced. Sprinkle with salt to taste.
4. Cook for 15 minutes until the vegetables are soft and gently browned. Cook for 20-25 minutes if you want crisper veggies.

5. When the vegetables are done, place them on a large serving dish. If necessary, season with more salt. Add a squeeze of fresh lime juice for extra flavor.
6. While the vegetable roast, bring a pot of water to a boil.
7. Put the hot water on the rice noodles. Soak for 6 to 10 minutes, or until the pasta is al dente - tender but still chewy and not overly soft. I usually find that 7 to 8 minutes is about right.
8. Rinse the soaked rice noodles under cold water quickly, shake, and set aside.
9. Soy sauce, sesame oil, maple syrup, balsamic vinegar, and garlic are mixed together to make the stir-fry sauce.
10. Heat a 12-inch large pan or wok over medium-high heat. Stir in the stir-fry sauce.
11. Add the rice noodles as soon as the sauce starts to boil.
12. Stir-fry the rice noodles for 1 minute, often tossing to coat and absorb the sauce.
13. Put the rice noodles in a serving bowl. Stir the noodles with the roasted veggies, or serve them separately in separate bowls.

154. BAKED SWEET POTATO

Prep Time: 5 Mins

Cook Time: 1 Hr

Total Time: 1 Hr 5 Mins

Servings: 2

Ingredients

- 2 medium sweet potatoes
- pinch of sea salt flakes
- 2 tsp olive oil

To serve

- butter, chili con carne, tuna mayo, baked beans, cheese, or green salad (optional)

Instructions

1. Set the oven to 180 degrees Celsius/160 degrees Celsius fan/gas 4. Scrub the sweet potatoes, place them on a baking sheet, and prick them all over with a fork. Drizzle a little oil over each and top with a pinch of sea salt flakes. Depending on size, bake for 45 to 1 hour, or until the exterior is crisp and easily pierced with a small knife. Add butter or your favorite filling to serve as a side dish.

155. BAKED SWEET POTATOES WITH GINGER AND HONEY

Prep Time: 15 Mins

Cook Time: 40 Mins

Total Time: 55 Mins

Servings: 12

Ingredients

- 3 pounds peeled and cubed sweet potatoes
- ½ cup of honey
- 3 tbsp grated fresh ginger
- 2 tbsp of walnut oil
- 1 tsp ground cardamom
- ½ tsp ground black pepper

Instructions

1. Preheat the oven to 400°F.
2. Toss the sweet potatoes, honey, ginger, walnut oil, cardamom, and pepper in a large mixing bowl. Transfer to a large cast-iron pan.
3. In a preheated oven, cook for 20 minutes. To release the pieces from the bottom of the pan, stir the potatoes. Cook for another 20 minutes until the sweet potatoes are soft and the exterior has caramelized.

156. BAKED BROWN RICE

Prep Time: 5 Mins

Cook Time: 1 Hr 5 Mins

Total Time: 1 Hr 10 Mins

Servings: 4

Ingredients

- 1 ½ cups of brown rice, medium or short grain
- 2 ½ cups of water
- 1 tbsp unsalted butter
- 1 tsp kosher salt

Instructions

1. Preheat the oven to 375 degrees Fahrenheit.
2. Put the rice in a square 8-inch glass baking dish.
3. Bring the water, butter, and salt to a boil in a kettle or covered saucepan. Pour the warm water over the rice, stir to mix, then cover securely with heavy-duty aluminum foil. Bake for 1 hour on the center rack of the oven.
4. Remove the cover after 1 hour and fluff the rice with a fork. Serve right away.

157. STIR-FRIED CURLY KALE WITH CHILLI & GARLIC

Prep Time: 5 Mins

Cook Time: 8 Mins

Servings: 4

Ingredients

- 1 tbsp olive oil
- 200g bag of curly kale
- 2 finely sliced garlic cloves
- 1 deseeded and sliced red chilli

Instructions

1. Warm the oil in a large wok, then add the kale and a couple tbsp of water. Season, then stir-fry for 5-8 minutes, adding the garlic and chili for the last 2 minutes. Take the kale from the fire when it is soft and vibrant green color, and serve.

158. ROAST BUTTERNUT SQUASH

Prep Time: 5 Mins

Cook Time: 45 Mins

Total Time: 50 Mins

Servings: 4

Ingredients

- 1 Butternut squash
- 2 tsp of olive oil
- Brown sugar, if desired
- salt and pepper to taste

Instructions

- Preheat the oven to 375 °F.
- Cut your butternut squash in half lengthwise with a large, sturdy knife.
- With a spoon, scoop out the seeds and stringy bits and discard or save for later (if roasting).
- Place the butternut squash, cut-side up, in a baking tray, and brush with olive oil or melted butter to coat the entire surface.
- Season to taste with salt, pepper, and brown sugar (if desired).
- It will take approximately 45 minutes in the oven, or until soft and fork-tender.
- Remove from the oven and cool. Scoop out the flesh and eat it plain or in your favorite recipes.

159. QUINOA STUFFED BELL PEPPERS

Prep Time: 20 Mins

Cook Time: 30 Mins

Total Time: 50 Mins

Servings: 6

Ingredients

- 3 cups of cooked quinoa
- 4-ounce green chiles
- 1 cup of corn kernels
- ½ cup of canned black beans, drained and rinsed
- ½ cup of petite diced tomatoes
- ½ cup of shredded Pepper Jack cheese
- ¼ cup of crumbled feta cheese
- 3 tbsp chopped fresh cilantro leaves
- 1 tsp cumin
- 1 tsp of garlic powder
- ½ tsp onion powder
- ½ tsp chili powder, or more to taste
- To taste, freshly ground black pepper and kosher salt
- 6 bell peppers, tops cut, stemmed, and seeded

Instructions

1. Preheat the oven to 350°F. Line a 9x13 baking sheet with parchment paper.
2. Mix quinoa, green chiles, corn, beans, tomatoes, cheeses, cilantro, cumin, garlic, onion, and chili powder in a large bowl. Season with salt and pepper to taste.
3. Fill each bell pepper cavity with the filling. Bake the filling in the oven sheet for 25 to 30 minutes, or until the peppers are tender.
4. Serve right away.

160. CARROT PILAF

Total Time: 30 Mins

Servings: 6

Ingredients

- 1 cup of shredded carrots
- ½ cup of chopped onion
- 1 tbsp butter
- 1 cup of uncooked long grain rice
- 14- ½ ounces of chicken broth
- 1 tsp lemon-pepper seasoning

Instructions

1. In a saucepan, sauté carrots and onion in butter until soft. Stir to coat the rice. Add the broth, lemon pepper, and stir. Bring to a boil. lower the heat, lid, and cook the rice for 20 minutes, or until it is soft.

161. QUINOA AND BLACK BEANS

Prep Time: 15 Mins

Cook Time: 35 Mins

Total Time: 50 Mins

Servings: 10

Ingredients

- 1 tsp vegetable oil
- 1 chopped onion
- 3 chopped garlic cloves
- ¾ cup of quinoa
- 1 ½ cups of vegetable broth
- 1 tsp of ground cumin
- ¼ tsp cayenne pepper
- salt and ground black pepper to taste

- 1 cup of frozen corn kernels
- 15-ounce black beans, rinsed and drained
- ½ cup of chopped fresh cilantro

Instructions

1. Simmer and stir the onion and garlic in a skillet over medium heat until gently browned, about 10 minutes.
2. Combine the quinoa with the onion mixture; pour the vegetable broth over; sprinkle with cumin, cayenne, salt, and pepper. Bring the mixture to a boil. Cover, lower the heat, and let it simmer for about 20 minutes, or until the quinoa is soft and the broth is gone.
3. Cook the frozen corn, stirring to combine, for about 5 minutes more, or until it is well heated through; stir in the black beans and cilantro.

162. SPRING ONION AND ZUCCHINI RIGATONI

Total Time: 30 Mins

Servings: 5

Ingredients

- 1 pound of rigatoni pasta
- 3 tbsp of olive oil
- 3 large minced garlic cloves
- 1 cup of thinly sliced red spring onions
- 3 medium zucchini, halved and thinly sliced
- ½ tsp red pepper flakes, or to taste
- ¼ cup of half and half
- To taste, add salt and freshly ground black pepper
- grated pecorino cheese, for topping

Instructions

1. Bring to a boil a big saucepan of salted water. Add the rigatoni, and cook it for around one minute less than the directions on the package, until it's just al dente (it will finish cooking at the end).
2. Meanwhile, in a big pan over medium-high heat, heat the olive oil. Add the garlic and red pepper flakes, and cook for 30 seconds, or until fragrant. Don't overcook or

you'll have mushy zucchini at the end. Add the onion and cook for 2 minutes until translucent. Add zucchini and cook for 3–4 minutes until just cooked.

3. Drain the pasta and mix it to the onion and zucchini. Add half-and-half and stir for a further 2 minutes, or until slightly thickened. Use salt and pepper to taste to season.

4. Divide among serving bowls and sprinkle with a lot of pecorino cheese, if you want. Serve warm.

163. BAKED PARMESAN YELLOW SQUASH ROUNDS

Prep Time: 5 Mins

Cook Time: 15 Mins

Total Time: 20 Mins

Servings: 4

Ingredients

- 2 medium-sized yellow summer squash
- Garlic salt & freshly ground black pepper
- ½ cup of freshly grated Parmesan cheese

Instructions

- Put an oven rack in the oven's center point. Set the oven to 425 °F. Line a baking sheet with foil or parchment paper (lightly sprayed with nonstick cooking spray).
- Wash and dry the squash before slicing it into ¼-inch thick slices. In the prepared pan, arrange the squash rounds with little to no space between them. Sprinkle the squash with a little freshly ground black pepper and garlic salt. Spread a thin coating of Parmesan cheese on each slice of squash with a small spoon.
- Bake the Parmesan for 15 to 20 minutes, or until it melts and turns a pale golden color. (Watch them carefully the first time you prepare them, and remove them from the oven early if the Parmesan is brown before 15 minutes.) To speed up the browning, broil them for a minute or two towards the end of the cooking time.) Serve right away.

164. RICE O'BRIEN

Total Time: 30 -60

Servings: 4

Ingredients

- 1 cup of long grain rice
- 1 large onion, chopped
- 1 tbsp soy sauce
- 1 large bell pepper, chopped
- 1 tsp salt
- ½ tsp poultry seasoning
- 2 ½ cups of chicken broth

Instructions

1. Combine rice, sliced onions, salt, poultry seasoning, soy sauce, finely chopped bell pepper, and chicken broth on a 2-quart baking sheet.

165. SPICY CHICKPEA DIP

Prep Time: 5 Mins

Cook Time: 10 Mins

Total Time: 15 Mins

Servings: 4

Ingredients

For the base

- 1 can of chickpeas
- 1 tbsp aquafaba
- 1 tsp ground cumin powder
- 3 cloves of garlic
- 1 tsp cilantro chopped finely, optional
- 1 jalapeno
- ½ tsp turmeric
- 2 tbsp divided olive oil
- 1 tsp red chili powder
- 1 tsp salt
- 1 tsp of lemon juice 1 tsp is approximately half a lemon

Instructions

2. Save 1 tbsp of the bringing juice from the chickpeas (aquafaba). Add a tbsp of water if you're using dried chickpeas.
3. Add a tsp of each turmeric, red chili powder, and cumin powder to a food processor along with the drained chickpeas, a couple of garlic cloves, one chopped jalapeno, and other ingredients. Pulse the ingredients in order to get a creamy mixture. Add approximately one tbsp of olive oil and continue pulsing.
4. Transfer to a bowl and top with cilantro and a tbsp of olive oil for a quick chickpea dip that the whole family will enjoy!

166. GREEK YOGURT DIP

Total Time: 5 Mins

Servings: 3

Ingredients

- 1 cup of yogurt plain full-fat
- ¼ tsp onion powder
- 1 tsp Olive Oil
- ¼ tsp garlic powder
- ¼ tsp Salt
- 1 tsp thyme
- 1 tsp Lime juice

Instructions

1. Mix together a cup of yogurt.
2. Mix garlic powder, onion powder, and thyme into the yogurt.
3. Then season with salt and pepper to taste. Add lime juice and olive oil. Mix all the ingredients until they become creamy.
4. Enjoy this creamy and healthy yogurt dip!

Notes

1. You may make this ahead of time and store it in the refrigerator for 3-4 days. Do not freeze.
2. Variations
3. Instead of using garlic powder, combine a freshly minced garlic clove with the thyme and onion.
4. To give this dip extra flavor, add chives, dried dill, or parsley.
5. Instead of using lime juice, use apple cider vinegar instead.
6. Using thick and creamy Greek yogurt, transform this dip into a greek yogurt dip.
7. Add some fresh jalapenos to this dip if you want to add some heat. The jalapenos must be finely minced in a food processor or blender before being added to the yogurt.

167. ROASTED GARLIC DIP

Prep Time: 15 Mins

Cook Time: 1 Hr

Additional: 2 Hrs 30 Mins

Total Time: 3 Hrs 45 Mins

Servings: 10

Ingredients

- 3 unpeeled heads of garlic
- 1 tbsp olive oil
- ½ cup of sour cream
- ¼ cup of mayonnaise
- 1 chopped green onions
- 1 tbsp red wine vinegar
- ½ tsp salt
- ¾ tbsp of ground black pepper

Instructions

1. Preheat the oven to 300 degrees Fahrenheit.
2. Cutting a ¼ inch from the top of each of the cloves will expose the garlic cloves. You may need to trim each clove along the sides of the head. Brush the sliced cloves with olive oil, then place the head in a piece of aluminum foil.
3. 1 hour in a preheated oven until the cloves are soft and well browned. Take it from the oven and allow it to cool to room temperature.
4. When the garlic cloves have cooled, squeeze them out of their skins and into a mixing bowl. A wire mixer thoroughly combines the sour cream, mayonnaise, green onions, vinegar, salt, and pepper. Stir until evenly combined, then place in the refrigerator for 2 to 4 hours to let the flavors to mix.

168. CRAB DELIGHT DIP

Total Time: 2 Hrs 5 Mins

Servings: 2 Cup

Ingredients

- 1 cup of mayonnaise
- 1 tbsp sherry wine
- ½ cup of sour cream
- 1 tsp lemon juice
- 6-ounce crabmeat
- salt and pepper

Instructions

1. Combine all of the ingredients.
2. Cool for at least 2 hours.
3. Serve with raw vegetables or crackers.

169. CARAMEL APPLE DIP

Total Time: 10 Mins

Servings: 10

Ingredients

- 1 ½ cups of heavy whipping cream
- ½ tsp ground cinnamon
- ½ tsp vanilla extract
- 1 tbsp granulated sugar
- ⅓ cup of caramel sauce, homemade or store-bought
- 4 ounces softened cream cheese, cut into pieces
- apple, sliced for serving

Instructions

1. In a stand mixer or large mixing bowl, smooth out the cream cheese. Add the cream and thoroughly combine for 3 minutes, or until stiff peaks form.
2. Add the sugar, caramel sauce, vanilla, cinnamon, and stir to mix.
3. Serve with slices of apple. Put leftovers in the fridge.

Notes

1. This dip is excellent to prepare ahead of time since it stays well for 5-7 days in the refrigerator. Before dipping, I prefer to let it thaw on the counter for a few minutes. For serving, slice the apples fresh, or toss them in with lemon juice to stop them from browning.

170. EASY CORNED BEEF DIP

Total Time: 10 Mins

Servings: 2 Cup

Ingredients

- 1 cup of diced corned beef
- 1 package dry onion soup mix
- 4 ounces of softened cream cheese, and cut into cubes
- 8 ounces sour cream
- 2 tbsp horseradish sauce
- crackers for dipping

Instructions

1. Combine the corned beef, onion soup, cream cheese, sour cream, and horseradish in a bowl. Mix well to incorporate all ingredients.
2. Refrigerate for at least 30 minutes and up to overnight.
3. Serve with crackers.
4. Keep leftover dip in the fridge in a covered container.

171. EASY SPINACH ARTICHOKE & SUN DRIED TOMATO DIP

Prep Time: 15 Mins

Cook Time: 25 Mins

Total Time: 40 Mins

Servings: 8

Ingredients

- 8-ounces of cream cheese
- ½ cup of plain Greek yogurt
- ½ cup of sour cream
- 1 8-ounce bag of fresh spinach
- 1 8.5 ounces can artichokes in brine, drained & chopped
- 1 8-ounce jar of sun-dried tomatoes in oil, drained & chopped
- ½ cup of shredded parmesan
- ½ cup of shredded mozzarella
- 4 minced cloves of garlic
- ½ tsp red pepper flakes (see notes)
- ½ tsp salt

Instructions

1. Spray some nonstick cooking spray on a baking dish and preheat your oven to 350 degrees.
2. Next, sauté your spinach over medium-high heat until it turns brilliant green and is slightly wilted. (2 to 3 minutes). Then move it to a bowl to chill. When the spinach is cool enough to handle, wrap it in a paper towel and squeeze out as much liquid as you can. Then cut it and put it in a big bowl.
3. Add the rest of your ingredients to the bowl and stir until everything is combined. Place your prepared baking dish with the dip ingredients in it, and cook for 20 to 25 minutes, or until the dip is hot and bubbly.
4. Serve right away with your preferred crackers.

Notes

1. Using ¼ tsp of red pepper flakes will make it not too spicy.

172. HOT BLT DIP

Prep Time: 10 Mins

Cook Time: 20 Mins

Total Time: 30 Mins

Servings: 20

Ingredients

- 1 pound of bacon, cooked and crumbled
- 1 cup of mayonnaise
- 1 cup of sour cream
- 8 ounces of softened cream cheese
- 1 ½ cups of shredded cheddar cheese
- 1 seeded and chopped tomato
- ¼ cup of sliced green onions
- Additional green onions, tomatoes, cooked bacon, and lettuce for garnish, if desired

Instructions

1. oven to 350 degrees Fahrenheit.
2. Thoroughly mix the cream cheese, mayonnaise, and sour cream in a bowl. Stir in the bacon crumbles to the mixture. Mix in the cheddar cheese, green onions, and tomatoes. Bake in a shallow dish or pie plate for 20 minutes or until bubbling. Add more tomatoes, green onions, and crumbled bacon as garnish. Serve with sliced baguettes or corn chips.

Notes

1. Make sure to squeeze the tomato to get rid of any extra juice before chopping it so that your dip doesn't have too much liquid.

173. BUFFALO CHICKEN DIP RECIPE

Prep Time: 10 Mins

Cook Time: 35 Mins

Total Time: 45 Mins

Servings: 12

Ingredients

- 3 large boiled and shredded boneless skinless chicken breasts
- 8 ounces of cubed cream cheese
- 1 cup of ranch dressing-homemade or store-bought
- 1 cup of hot sauce, plus more as needed
- 1 tsp freshly ground black pepper
- 1 tsp of garlic powder
- ½ cup of chopped green onion
- 1.5 cups of mozzarella cheese-shredded, divided
- 1.5 cups of cheddar cheese-shredded, divided

Instructions

2. Cook the chicken. If your chicken isn't cooked through, bring a large pot of water to a boil over high heat. Add the chicken breasts and heat the saucepan back to a boil. Remove it from the heat and cover it with a tight-fitting lid. Allow your chicken to poach, covered, for around 25 minutes. Remove from the saucepan when thoroughly cooked and let stand until cool enough to handle (note-the cooking time for the chicken is not included in the total cooking time for this dish).
3. Prep. Spray non-stick cooking spray in a 9x9-inch baking pan (or a pan that approximates that size) and preheat your oven to 350 degrees F.
4. Heat the sauce. Add the cubed cream cheese, ranch dressing, spicy sauce, black pepper, and garlic powder to a medium saucepot set over medium-low heat. Constantly mix until the cream cheese is completely dissolved in the ranch and spicy sauce. removing the heat.
5. Combine. Add 1 cup of shredded mozzarella cheese, 1 cup of shredded cheddar cheese, green onion, cooked and shredded chicken, and sauce to the pot. Mix well. Transfer to the prepared baking pan and top with the remaining mozzarella and cheddar cheese.

6. Bake. Bake for about 20–30 minutes, or until the cheese is melted and the edges are bubbling. Set the oven to broil. Until the top of your buffalo chicken dip is golden brown, allow it another 2-3 minutes to cook. Remove it right away.
7. Serve. Serve with crackers, veggie sticks, tortilla chips, or leftovers wrapped in a tortilla with your favorite greens.

Notes

1. The approximately 30-minute cooking time for the chicken is not included in the total cooking time. If you're short on time, I advise making the chicken ahead of time.
2. About 4 cups of shredded rotisserie chicken can bc used as a substitution.
3. Use your favorite blue cheese dressing or ranch dressing.
4. Grate your cheese. When compared to pre-shredded, packaged cheese, freshly shredded cheese always comes together better.
5. If you want to add a more pungent cheese, try Jack cheese, blue cheese crumbles, or feta cheese.
6. For around 2 or 3 days, leftovers taste lovely. Reheat in the microwave or in an oven preheated to 350°F and tented with foil.
7. This recipe is simple to make in a crockpot. The only difference is that the cheese on top of the Crock-Pot version won't be brown and bubbly.

174. COWBOY DIP RECIPE

Total Time: 10 Mins

Servings: 8

Ingredients

- 1 ½ cups of sour cream
- 2 tbsp Ranch Dressing Mix
- 3 tbsp of cooked and crumbled bacon
- 1 cup of shredded cheddar cheese
- ½ tsp garlic salt
- 3 tsp horseradish
- 1 tsp Worcestershire sauce
- 1 tbsp green onions sliced

Instructions

1. In a medium bowl, mix the bacon bits, ranch dressing mix, sour cream, cheddar cheese, garlic salt, horseradish, and Worcestershire sauce.
2. As a garnish, sprinkle the green onions on top.
3. Serve with veggies, chips, or slices of pita bread.

Notes

1. If you want to cut calories, try replacing the sour cream with plain Greek yogurt: Greek yogurt and sour cream taste almost the same to me.

175. JALAPEÑO POPPER DIP

Prep Time: 10 Mins

Cook Time: 15 Mins

Total Time: 25 Mins

Servings: 12

Ingredients

- 4 ounces diced jalapenos, well-drained (include seeds if you like it really spicy)
- 8 ounces of softened cream cheese
- 1 cup of sour cream
- 1 tsp of garlic powder
- 2 cups of shredded cheddar cheese
- ¾ cup of shredded parmesan cheese

Topping

- 1 cup of Panko bread crumbs
- 4 tbsp melted butter or margarine
- ¼ cup of shredded parmesan cheese
- 1 tbsp fresh parsley

Instructions

2. Heat the oven to 375°F.

3. Mix cream cheese, garlic powder, and sour cream in a mixing bowl on medium speed until fluffy.
4. Mix in the cheddar cheese, ¾ cup of parmesan cheese, and diced jalapenos.
5. Spread into an 8x8 baking sheet.
6. Mix together bread crumbs, melted butter, ¼ cup of shredded parmesan cheese, and parsley.
7. Crumble the crumb topping on top of the cream cheese mixture.
8. Cook for 15-20 minutes until the breadcrumbs are golden brown.

176. FRENCH ONION DIP

Prep Time: 5 Mins

Cook Time: 5 Mins

Chilling Time: 1 Hr

Total Time: 1 Hr 10 Mins

Servings: 12

Ingredients

- 2 cups of sour cream
- 2 tbsp of dried chopped onions
- 2 tsp of onion powder
- ⅛ tsp of garlic powder
- ½ tsp kosher salt
- 2 tsp of dried parsley
- 2 tsp better than bouillon beef

Instructions

1. Stir together the sour cream, chopped onions, onion powder, garlic powder, salt, parsley, and better than bouillon beef in a medium mixing bowl.
2. Refrigerate the dip for an hour to allow the flavors to blend.

177. LOADED BAKED POTATO DIP

Prep Time: 15 Mins

Chilling Time: 1 Hr

Total Time: 1 Hr 15 Mins

Servings: 10

Ingredients

- 5 strips of center-cut bacon
- 1 small finely chopped jalapeno pepper, optional
- 8 ounces of full-fat cream cheese
- 1 cup of sour cream
- 1-ounce ranch seasoning and dressing mix, dry (do not prepare)
- 1½ cups of extra-sharp Cheddar cheese, freshly grated
- ¼ cup of thinly sliced green onions
- ½ tsp freshly cracked pepper

What to dip in it:

- Thick potato chips with ridges or pretzel crisps
- Celery sticks

Instructions

1. Bacon: Cook the bacon strips in a pan over medium heat until crispy. Alternatively, use pre-cooked bacon and heat it as per package directions. Baked bacon is another option. Put the bacon on a plate that's been lined with paper towels, and use the towels to soak up any extra oil that's on the plate. Chop coarsely and set aside.
2. Take the jalapeno's seeds out and cut it into thin slices.
3. Cream cheese Place an unwrapped block of cream cheese on a microwave-safe plate. Microwave for 15-20 seconds, then remove and flip over for another 10 seconds if necessary.
4. Using an electric hand mixer, smooth up the softened cream cheese. Mix the sour cream and DRY ranch mix (do not prepare the mix.) Stir in the sliced Cheddar cheese, green onions, chopped jalapeno, and freshly cracked pepper until mixed. If you want your bacon to stay crisp, stir it in here (it will soften) or top the dip with it.
5. Chill: Refrigerate the dip for an hour or so before serving if you have time. It's delicious straight away and much better after chilling.

6. Serve the dip in a bowl with your favorite sturdy potato chips. Serve the dip with a table knife on the side; because the dip is thick and easily breaks the chips, scraping from the dip with a knife is easier. Pretzel chips and celery sticks work well in this dip as well.

7. Refrigerate any leftovers in a sealed jar for up to 1 week. Because of the dairy content, this dip should not be left at room temperature for more than 2 hours.

Notes

1. This dip is mostly salty. There is a good amount of salt between the ranch dip, the bacon, and the potato chips.

178. GREEK LAYERED HUMMUS DIP

Prep Time: 15 Mins

Total Time: 15 Mins

Servings: 8

Ingredients

- 17-ounce container of prepared hummus
- 1 ½ cup of plain Greek yogurt
- ½ cup of English cucumber pieces
- ¼ cup of chopped roasted red peppers
- ¼ cup of chopped pitted kalamata olives
- 1 tbsp of olive oil, plus additional for drizzling
- ¼ cup of diced red onion
- 1 tbsp of freshly chopped parsley leaves
- ¼ tsp salt
- 1 ounce of crumbled feta cheese
- 2 tbsp toasted pine nuts
- ½ tsp of fresh ground black pepper
- **Serving suggestions**
- Cucumber slices
- pita bread, pita wedges
- carrots

- use as a spread on sandwiches
- celery
- crackers

Instructions

1. Pour the hummus onto a small serving plate. Dollop the yogurt on top and then carefully spread it to cover the hummus, leaving a border showing through.
2. Mix the cucumber, peppers, olives, onion, 1 tbsp olive oil, parsley, salt, and pepper in a small bowl. Pour the vegetable mixture evenly over the yogurt. Top the vegetables with crumbled feta cheese and toasted pine nuts. Drizzle a little extra olive oil over the dip. Serve right away.

Notes

1. Roasted red peppers should be available on the olive bar at your local grocery store, but jarred works just as well.
2. For the best presentation, serve this Greek Layered Hummus Dip right away after assembling it.
3. Up to 24 hours of dip can be stored in an airtight container. Smear leftovers on regular sandwiches for a delicious flavor boost.

179. HOT BACON CHEESY DIP RECIPE

Prep Time: 10 Mins

Cook Time: 20 Mins

Servings: 2 Cup

Ingredients

- 8- ounce soft cream cheese
- 2 cups of shredded cheddar cheese
- 8- ounce Greek yogurt
- ¼ cup of mayonnaise
- 6 slices bacon cooked crisp and chopped
- 1 tbsp Worcestershire sauce
- ¼ tsp red pepper
- ¼ tsp onion powder

Instructions

1. Combine all ingredients except the ¼ cup of cheddar cheese and ¼ cup of bacon in a bowl.
2. Spread the mixture in a 2-cup of oven-safe container.
3. Top with the remaining cheese and bacon.
4. Bake at 350°F for 18–20 minutes, or until hot and bubbly.
5. Serve with chips, crackers, or veggies.

180. CHEESY TEXAS TRASH DIP

Total Time: 25 Mins

Servings: 8 Cups

Ingredients

- 1 8-ounce package of cream cheese
- 1 7-ounce can of sliced green chiles, drained
- 1 cup of sour cream
- 2 16-ounce cans of refried beans
- 1 package Taco Seasoning Mix
- 4 cups of shredded Mexican cheese blend, divided
- green onion, chopped for serving
- Sliced black olives for serving

Instructions

1. Heat the oven to 350°F. Microwave cream cheese and sour cream in a large microwaveable bowl for 1 minute on high or until softened. Remove from the microwave. Mix with a wire whisk until smooth. Mix in the refried beans, green chiles, seasoning mix, and 2 cups of cheese.
2. Spread the bean mixture onto a 13x9-inch baking sheet that has been sprayed with nonstick cooking spray. Top with the remaining 2 cups of cheese.
3. Bake for 25 minutes or until the cheese has melted. Garnish with green onion and black olives, if desired. Serve alongside tortilla chips.

181. SPINACH DIP

Prep Time: 10 Mins

Cook Time: 20 Mins

Total Time: 30 Mins

Servings: 10

Ingredients

- 8 ounces of softened cream cheese
- 1 cup of sour cream
- 10 ounces of fresh spinach leaves
- 1 tsp minced garlic
- ½ tsp salt
- ¼ tsp pepper
- ½ cup of grated parmesan cheese
- 1 ½ cups of shredded mozzarella cheese divided use
- 1 tbsp chopped parsley
- bread, crackers, and vegetables for serving
- cooking spray

Instructions

1. Sauté or steam the spinach until it has wilted. Allow to cool, then squeeze out all extra water. Chop the spinach coarsely.
2. Preheat the oven to 375 degrees Fahrenheit. Cooking spray a small baking sheet or pan.
3. In a mixing bowl, combine the cream cheese, sour cream, cooked spinach, garlic, salt, pepper, parmesan cheese, and ¾ cup of mozzarella cheese. Stir until well mixed.
4. Fill the prepared pan with the spinach mixture. Finish with the remaining mozzarella cheese.
5. Bake for 20 minutes until the cheese has melted and the dip is boiling. Cook for another 2-3 minutes, or until the cheese starts to brown, on broil.
6. Garnish with parsley and serve with bread, crackers, and veggies.

182. ZUCCHINI LASAGNA RECIPE

Prep Time: 30 Mins

Cook Time: 50 Mins

Total Time: 1 Hr 20 Mins

Servings: 12

Ingredients

- 4 large zucchinis
- 2 pounds of ground beef
- 24-ounces of pasta sauce
- 15-ounce ricotta cheese
- 1 cup of shredded parmesan regianno
- 1 ½ cups of mozzarella
- salt and pepper
- 1 egg
- small handful fresh parsley and basil chopped

Instructions

1. Preheat the oven to 400 degrees Fahrenheit.
2. Cut the zucchini into thin slices, as thin or thick as you like. Place aside.
3. In a large skillet over medium-high heat, brown the ground meat. With a spatula, finely break down the ground beef and pan fry it until browned and no longer pink.
4. Pour the pasta sauce over the ground beef (reserve ½ cup), stir well, and remove from heat.
5. Make the ricotta mix in a medium mixing bowl by mixing the ricotta cheese, parmesan, egg, salt, and pepper.
6. Cover the bottom of a 9x13-inch casserole dish with ½ cup of pasta sauce.
7. Place the zucchini pieces on top of the pasta sauce. You may overlap them or place them side by side.
8. Top the zucchini with half of the bolognese sauce and half of the ricotta mixture.
9. On top of the ricotta, put ½ cup of grated mozzarella along with chopped parsley and basil.

10. Repeat these layers a final time.
11. Finish with a final layer of zucchini slices, chopped parsley and basil, and ½ cup of mozzarella cheese.
12. Cook the lasagna for 40-45 minutes in the oven. For a nice golden top, broil for a couple of minutes.
13. Serve garnished with whole basil leaves.

183. ROASTED RATATOUILLE QUINOA

Prep Time: 10 Mins

Cook Time: 25-30 Mins

Total Time: 35-40 Mins

Servings: 4

Ingredients

- ¼ tsp dried rosemary
- ¼ tsp dried thyme
- ½ tsp dried oregano
- ¼ tsp garlic powder
- Pinch of red pepper flakes
- 1 tsp kosher salt
- ½ tsp black pepper
- 2 tbsp of olive oil
- 4 medium zucchini, cut into ½ -inch dice
- 2 medium eggplants, cut into ½ -inch dice
- 1-pint cherry or grape tomatoes
- 2 red bell peppers, cut into ½ -inch dice
- Half an onion, cut into ½ -inch dice
- ½ cup of quinoa
- 1 cup of water
- 1 tbsp chopped basil

Instructions

1. Preheat the oven to 400 degrees Fahrenheit.

2. Mix the rosemary, thyme, oregano, garlic powder, red pepper flakes, salt, and pepper in a small bowl.
3. Stir the zucchini, squash, and eggplant with 1 tbsp olive oil and half of the dry seasoning mix on a baking sheet. Spread it out in a single layer.
4. Stir the tomatoes, peppers, and red onions with 1 tbsp olive oil and the remaining dried spice mix on another sheet pan. Spread it out in a single layer.
5. Roast for 25-30 minutes until the zucchini, squash, and eggplant are lightly browned, the tomatoes and peppers are wrinkled, and the onions are translucent.
6. Make the quinoa on the burner while the vegetable roast. Mix the quinoa and water in a small saucepan over high heat. Bring to a boil, then lower to low heat and cook for 10-12 minutes, or until the grains are cooked. Allow for a 5-minute rest before fluffing with a fork.
7. Combine the roasted veggies, quinoa, and basil in a large bowl.

184. GIANT BUTTER BEAN STEW

Prep Time: 30 Mins

Cook Time: 1 Hr 15 Mins

Total Time: 1 Hr 45 Mins

Servings: 6

Ingredients

- 4 x 235g cans butter beans (cook according to pack instructions)
- 3 small finely sliced red onions
- 100ml Greek extra virgin olive oil
- 2 large finely sliced carrots
- 3 finely chopped celery stalks with leaves
- 4 sliced sundried tomatoes
- 1kg ripe tomatoes, skinned, deseeded, and finely chopped
- 4 chopped garlic cloves
- 1 tsp paprika
- 1 tsp ground cinnamon
- 2 tbsp tomato purée
- 1 tsp sugar
- small pack flat-leaf parsley, finely chopped

- small pack of dill, finely chopped
- 100g crumbled feta (optional)

Instructions

1. Reserve 200ml of the liquid from the canned beans. Cook the onions, carrots, and celery in a large flameproof lidded casserole dish until tender and until the onions are soft and translucent but not colored. Stir in the other ingredients, reserving half of the herbs and feta for garnish (if using).
2. Heat oven to 180° Celsius/160° Celsius fan/gas 4. Cook for 5 minutes on low heat, then pour in the reserved liquid. Cover the bowl and bake for 40 minutes. Check periodically to ensure the beans are not drying out; if necessary, add a bit more water.
3. Remove the lid and bake for another 10 minutes. Can be made ahead of time and reheated. Just before serving, crumble the remaining feta over the top and season with salt and pepper to you taste.

185. STUFFED EGGPLANT

Prep Time: 30 Mins

Cook Time: 50 Mins

Total Time: 1 Hr 20 Mins

Servings: 4

Ingredients

- 1 large eggplant
- 3 tbsp extra-virgin olive oil
- ½ tsp grey sea salt
- ¼ tsp black pepper
- ½ pound ground beef
- 1 diced small onion
- 1 small diced red bell pepper
- 3 finely chopped cloves garlic
- ½ cup of chopped fresh parsley
- ½ cup of chopped fresh basil leaves
- 1 ¼ cups of grated pecorino Romano cheese

- ½ cup of plain panko crispy bread crumbs
- 1 whole egg
- 2 small chopped tomatoes

Instructions

1. Preheat the oven to 350°F.
2. Take out the eggplant's center, leaving enough meat inside the skin since it will hold its shape when cooked. Cut the scooped-out eggplant; place in a pot, cover with water and cook until very soft, 10 to 12 minutes.
3. Meanwhile, in a medium sauté pan over medium heat, heat 1 tbsp olive oil. Season the beef with salt and pepper. Sauté the seasoned ground beef in the pan until all of the liquid has evaporated and the beef has begun to color slightly. Let the cooked beef cool for a few minutes, then chop it up, so there are no big chunks of meat. In the leftover 2 tbsp of olive oil, sauté the onion, pepper, and garlic over medium heat.
4. Combine the cooked eggplant, veggies, meat, herbs, 1 cup of cheese, ¼ cup of the bread crumbs, and the egg in a mixing bowl. Pour this mixture into the two sides of the scooped eggplants, evenly dividing it.
5. Add salt and pepper and top with sliced tomatoes, the remaining ¼ cup of cheese, and the remaining ¼ cup of bread crumbs. Bake for 50 minutes on an oiled oven tray or baking dish. Briefly cool; slice widthwise and serve.

186. SAUTÉED CABBAGE

Prep Time: 5 Mins

Cook Time: 10 Mins

Total Time: 15 Mins

Servings: 6

Ingredients

- 1 small head of green cabbage
- 1 tbsp extra virgin olive oil
- 1 tbsp unsalted butter
- 1 ½ tsp kosher salt
- ½ tsp freshly ground black pepper
- 1 tbsp chopped fresh thyme optional
- ½ tbsp of apple cider vinegar plus more to taste

Instructions

1. Cut the cabbage in half from the top to the core. Place them on your cutting board and slice them as thinly as possible around the core to create fine ribbons. Remove the core.
2. Over medium-high heat, heat a large sauté pan or similar heavy-bottomed pot. Add the olive oil and butter. Add the salt, cabbage, and pepper when the butter has melted. Cook, occasionally stirring, for 10-15 minutes, or until the cabbage is soft and starting to brown. You don't need to stir it constantly. Allowing cabbage to sit undisturbed for a minute or two will allow it to develop caramelized brown pieces (aka FLAVOR).
3. Add apple cider vinegar and take of heat. If you want to add more zingy and acidic flavors, you may taste the recipe and add a little extra salt, pepper, or vinegar. Garnish with thyme. Serve hot.

Notes

1. Refrigerate sautéed cabbage for up to one week in an airtight jar for up to one week.
2. Reheat sautéed cabbage in a microwave-safe bowl or on a plate until warm. After reheating, add another pinch of salt and a splash of apple cider vinegar to your leftovers.
3. If frozen in a freezer-safe container, sautéed cabbage can be frozen. The cabbage may change a little in texture while it's frozen, but it will still taste great when it's thawed.

187. BASIC SAUTÉED KALE

Total Time: 25 Mins

Servings: 4

Ingredients

- 1 tbsp plus 1 tsp of extra-virgin olive oil, divided
- 1-1 ½ pound of kale, ribs removed, coarsely chopped
- ½ cup of water
- 2 minced garlic cloves
- ¼ tsp crushed red pepper
- 2-3 tsp sherry vinegar or red-wine vinegar
- ¼ tsp salt

Instructions

1. In a Dutch oven, heat 1 tbsp of oil over medium heat. Cook, stirring with two big spoons until the kale is brilliant green, around 1 minute. Reduce the heat to the medium-low, lid, and cook for 12 to 15 minutes, or until the kale is soft. Push the kale to one side and sauté the garlic and crushed red pepper in the remaining 1 tsp oil until fragrant, 30 seconds to 1 minute. Remove from the heat and stir everything together. Add salt and vinegar to taste.

188. SAUTEED KALE WITH APPLES

Prep Time: 15 Mins

Cook Time: 15 Mins

Total Time: 30 Mins

Servings: 4

Ingredients

- 1 tbsp olive oil
- 1 sliced white onion
- 2 Red Delicious apples, peeled and cored, sliced into bite-size pieces
- 2 tsp apple cider vinegar
- ⅛ tsp sea salt
- ⅛ tsp ground black pepper
- 4 cups of chopped kale leaves

Instructions

2. Bring the olive oil to heat in a pan over medium heat; sauté and stir the onion until tender, approximately 4 minutes. Add apples, vinegar, salt, and pepper to a pan; cover and heat for 3 minutes, or until apples are soft. Cover and boil until the kale is soft, 4 to 5 minutes.

189. ROASTED BEETS AND SAUTEED BEET GREENS

Cook Time: 1 Hr

Total Time: 1 Hr 10 Mins

Servings: 4

Ingredients

- 1 bunch of beets with
- greens
- ¼ cup of divided olive oil
- 2 minced garlic cloves
- 2 tbsp of chopped onion (Optional)
- salt and pepper to taste
- 1 tbsp red wine vinegar (Optional)

Instructions

1. Preheat the oven to 350°F. Remove the leaves and thoroughly wash the beets, leaving the skins on. Rinse the greens, remove any big stems, and set them aside. Mix the beets with 2 tbsp of olive oil in a small baking sheet or roasting pan. If you choose to peel the beets, it is better to do so after roasting them.
2. Simmer for 45–60 minutes, or until a knife easily slides through the largest beet.
3. When the roasted beets are almost done, heat the remaining 2 tbsp olive oil in a pan over medium-low heat. Cook the garlic and onion for 1 minute. Tear the beet greens into 2 to 3-inch pieces and add them to the skillet. Cook, often stirring, until the greens are wilted and soft. Season with salt and pepper to taste. Serve the greens plain and the roasted beets sliced with red wine vinegar, butter, salt, and pepper.

190. GREEK BROWN RICE AND VEGETABLE CASSEROLE

Prep Time: 30 Mins

Cook Time: 1 Hr 30 Mins

Total Time: 2 Hrs 40 Mins

Servings 8

Ingredients

- 2 tbsp of olive oil, plus additional for oiling the baking dish
- 1 medium chopped onion
- 2 medium chopped red bell peppers
- 1 medium chopped yellow bell pepper
- 2 medium zucchini halved lengthwise and sliced into half-moons
- 1 medium yellow squash halved lengthwise and cut into half-moons
- 4 chopped garlic cloves
- ¼ cup of chopped fresh parsley divided
- 1 tbsp chopped fresh oregano
- 1 tbsp chopped fresh dill
- ½ tsp crushed red pepper flakes, optional
- 4 cups of cooked brown rice
- 1 cup of ricotta cheese, light is fine
- 1 cup of crumbled feta cheese is reduced fat or fat-free is fine
- 1 large egg
- 2 tbsp of lemon juice
- to taste, salt and freshly ground black pepper
- ¼ cup of pitted and halved Kalamata olives
- 2 medium tomatoes

Instructions

1. Preheat the oven to 375°F. Grease a 13 x 9-inch baking sheet lightly. Place aside.
2. Heat the oil to medium-high. Simmer for 4-5 minutes, or until the onion begins to soften.
3. Cook for 5-6 minutes, or until the bell pepper begins to soften.
4. Cook for 3-4 minutes more, or until the zucchini and yellow squash begins to soften.
5. If using, stir in the garlic, 2 tbsp minced parsley, oregano, dill, and crushed red pepper flakes. Allow cooling slightly.

6. Combine veggies, brown rice, ricotta and feta cheeses, egg, lemon juice, and salt and black pepper to taste in a large bowl. Smooth the top of the prepared baking sheet.
7. Sprinkle with half Kalamata olives and tomato slices on top.
8. Bake for 45 minutes to 1 hour, or until heated all the way through.
9. Remove from the oven and top with the remaining chopped parsley.

Notes

1. Cooking the brown rice is not included in the prep time. I like to prepare a big batch and freeze it so that I always have it on hand.

Substitutions

2. Ricotta can be substituted with pureed cottage cheese or silken tofu.
3. Although the casserole will not have the same Greek flavor, mozzarella or Monterey jack will work.
4. Quinoa can be substituted for brown rice.

191. SIMPLE LEMON-HERB CHICKEN

Prep Time: 10 Mins

Cook Time: 15 Mins

Total Time: 25 Mins

Servings: 2

Ingredients

- 5-ounce skinless, boneless chicken breast halves
- 1 medium lemon
- salt and ground black pepper to taste
- 1 tbsp olive oil
- 1 pinch of dried oregano
- 2 sprigs of fresh parsley for garnish

Instructions

1. Cut the lemon in halves and strain ½ lemon juice over the chicken. Season with salt to taste. Allow it to sit while heating the oil in a small skillet over medium-low heat.

2. When the oil is heated, add the chicken to the skillet. Add the juice from the other ½ lemon, pepper to taste, and oregano to the chicken as it cooks. Cook each side for 5 to 10 minutes, or until the juices run clear. Garnish with parsley if desired.

192. GRILLED LEMON CHICKEN

Prep Time: 10 Mins

Cook Time: 15 Mins

Marinating Time: 30 Mins

Total Time: 55 Mins

Servings: 6

Ingredients

- 6 6 ounces boneless skinless chicken breasts
- ¼ cup of olive oil
- ¼ cup of lemon juice plus the zest of the lemons
- ½ tsp salt
- 2 tsp oregano
- 4 garlic cloves pressed
- ¼ tsp black pepper
- parsley or cilantro for serving
- lemon wedges for serving

Instructions

1. If some parts of the chicken are too thick, pat it dry and pound it. In a bowl or resealable freezer bag, combine the olive oil, lemon juice, oregano, garlic, salt, and pepper. Toss in the chicken and toss well to mix. Allow at least 30 minutes to marinate.
2. Preheat the grill or grill pan to medium-high. Grill, the chicken for 5-7 minutes on each side. Flip with tongs and cook until juices run dry, about 5-7 minutes longer. Discard excess marinade
3. Take the chicken off the grill. If desired, garnish with parsley and serve with lemon wedges and veggies.

1. Storage Keep any leftovers in an airtight container. They can last up to four days.

193. HOME-STYLE CHICKEN CURRY

Prep Time: 15 Mins

Cook Time: 30 Mins

Total Time: 45 Mins

Servings: 4

Ingredients

- 1 large onion
- 6 roughly chopped garlic cloves
- 50g roughly chopped ginger
- 4 tbsp vegetable oil
- 2 tsp cumin seeds
- 1 tsp fennel seeds
- 5cm cinnamon stick
- 1 tsp chili flakes
- 1 tsp garam masala
- 1 tsp turmeric
- 1 tsp caster sugar
- 400g can of chopped tomatoes
- 8 chicken thighs, skinned, boneless
- 250ml of hot chicken stock
- 2 tbsp chopped coriander

Instructions

1. 1 big onion, roughly chopped, in a small food processor with 3 tbsp water, processed to a slack paste. You may use a stick blender for this or coarsely grate the onion into a bowl—no need to add water if grating the onion. Place it in a small bowl and set it aside.
2. In the same food processor, combine 6 roughly chopped garlic cloves and 50g of roughly chopped ginger with 4 tbsp of water; process until smooth and transfer into

another small bowl. Alternatively, finely grate the ginger and smash the garlic to a paste using a knife or garlic press.

3. Warm 4 tbsp of vegetable oil in a wok or large pan over medium heat.
4. Add 2 tsp cumin seeds, 1 tsp fennel seeds, a 5 cm cinnamon stick, and 1 tsp chilli flakes all at once to the pan. Swirl everything together for about 30 seconds, or until the spices release an aromatic aroma.
5. Add the onion paste; it will sputter at first. Sauté until the water evaporates and the onions have turned a lovely dark golden color, around 7-8 minutes.
6. Cook for another 2 minutes, stirring frequently, after adding the garlic and ginger paste.
7. Cook for 20 seconds after adding 1 tsp garam masala, 1 tsp turmeric, and 1 tsp caster sugar before adding a 400g can chopped tomatoes.
8. Cook for approximately ten minutes on medium heat, without a lid, until the tomatoes decrease and color.
9. Once the tomatoes have thickened to a paste, add 8 skinless, boneless chicken thighs in 3 cm chunks to the pan.
10. Cook for 5 minutes to cover the chicken in the masala and lock in the juices, then add in 250ml of boiling chicken stock.
11. Simmer without a cover for 8–10 minutes, or until the chicken is soft and the masala has gently thickened—you may need to add an extra ladleful of stock or water if the curry needs it.
12. Serve with 2 tbsp of chopped coriander and Indian flatbreads or fluffy basmati rice, as well as a pot of yogurt on the side.

194. BOILED CHICKEN AND RICE RECIPE

Prep Time: 10 Mins

Cook Time: 1 Hr 30 Mins

Total Time: 1 Hr 40 Mins

Servings: 12

Ingredients

- 1 medium chicken
- water
- 2-3 cups of long grain rice
- 1 tbsp salt
- 1 tsp pepper
- 1 lime optional

Instructions

1. Add the chicken to the stockpot. Place the chicken in a large stockpot. Cover the chicken with water up to the top. Simmer for 1–1.5 hours, covered.
2. To remove the chicken, use tongs (keep the broth in the pot). Place the chicken in a large mixing bowl. Remove the chicken meat and shred it. Return the shredded chicken to the pot. 2 cups of rice, salt, and pepper. Simmer for about 15 minutes (or per package instructions). If the soup is too soupy, add extra rice halfway through.
3. Serve. Serve warm with a squeeze of lime juice and freshly cracked black pepper.

Notes

1. Swap the whole chicken with chicken breasts. Cook for 15 minutes in 4-6 cups of chicken broth for boneless chicken breasts and 30 minutes for bone-in chicken breasts.
2. Refrigerate for up to five days, or frozen for up to three months.
3. Freeze in single or family portions if freezing. When ready to serve, defrost overnight and cook on the stovetop.
4. Serve as is or with your favorite steamed.

195. SIMPLE ROASTED BUTTERNUT SQUASH

Prep Time: 15 Mins

Cook Time: 25 Mins

Total Time: 40 Mins

Servings: 4

Ingredients

- 1 butternut squash—peeled, seeded, and cut into 1-inch cubes
- 2 tbsp of olive oil
- 2 cloves of garlic, minced
- salt and ground black pepper to taste

Instructions

1. Preheat the oven to 400°F.
2. Combine butternut squash, olive oil, and garlic in a large mixing bowl. Season with salt and black pepper to taste. Arrange the coated squash on a baking tray.
3. Roast in a preheated oven for 25 to 30 minutes, or until the squash is soft and lightly browned.

196. BEST CHICKEN AND RICE

Prep Time: 20 Mins

Cook Time: 45 Mins

Total Time: 1 Hr 5 Mins

Servings: 5

Ingredients

Chicken

- 5 chicken thighs, skin-on and bone-in
- 2 tbsp of olive oil

Marinade

- 2 lemons juiced and zested (approx. ¼ cup of juice)
- 2 tsp Dijon Mustard
- 3 garlic cloves minced
- 1 tsp dried oregano
- 1 tsp dried thyme
- ½ tsp salt
- ¼ tsp black pepper
- 1 tbsp olive oil

Rice

- 1 yellow onion diced
- 2 cups of baby spinach lightly packed and roughly chopped
- 2 garlic cloves minced
- 1 tsp dried oregano
- 1 cup of long grain white rice
- 2 cups of chicken stock
- ½ tsp salt
- ¼ tsp black pepper
- chopped parsley for garnish
- Lemon zest or slices for garnish

Instructions

1. Marinate the chicken.
2. In a bowl, mix all marinade ingredients.
3. Put the chicken thighs in a glass dish, pour the marinade over them, and turn to coat. Refrigerate the chicken for at least 30 minutes and up to overnight in a covered bowl.
4. Prepare the chicken and rice.
5. Set the oven to 350° Fahrenheit. 2 tbsp olive oil, heated in a large ovenproof skillet over medium-high heat Cook until the skin on the chicken thighs is golden brown, about 5 minutes. Save any leftover marinade for later use.
6. Cook for about 5 minutes on the other side. Set aside the chicken thighs from the skillet.
7. Scrape and remove any browned bits with tongs, then gather a couple of paper towels to soak up some, but not all, of the fat from the pan. Keep a little grease to cook the onions.
8. Stir in the chopped onions for 1-2 minutes or until they begin to become translucent.
9. Combine the chopped spinach, garlic, oregano, salt, pepper, and leftover marinade in a mixing bowl. Stir for 30 seconds more, or until the spinach begins to wilt.
10. Stir the rice in the skillet to evenly coat it with the oil.
11. Pour in the chicken stock and mix to combine. On the burner, bring this to a simmer.
12. Place the chicken thighs on top of the rice, then cover and bake in the preheated oven. Cook for 35 minutes. Take the lid, return the skillet to the oven, and bake until the chicken is cooked through and the rice is tender, about 10 minutes more.
13. Allow 5 to 10 minutes for the chicken and rice to rest. As the spinach and onions rise to the top, the rice will look very dark. Before serving, fluff the rice with a fork to bring everything back together.
14. Garnish with parsley and grilled lemon slices or fresh lemon zest.

Notes

1. **To store:** Any leftover chicken may be refrigerated in an airtight container for three to four days.
2. **To freeze:** Place any leftovers in a freezer-safe container and freeze for up to 2 months.
3. **For reheating:** Cook the chicken for 2 to 3 minutes in the microwave. Run the chicken under the broiler for a few minutes to crisp up the skin. Watch it closely to ensure that it does not burn.

THE END

Made in the USA
Monee, IL
24 April 2023

32328292R00116